Quality Control and Regulatory Aspects for Biologicals

This book serves as a comprehensive guide on quality control and regulatory aspects for biological products. It covers a wide range of topics, including regulatory requirements, quality control strategies, analytical methods, and risk management. It delves into the advantages and limitations of in vivo tests and discusses alternative methods that can be employed. The book explores the use of animal-based testing methods in quality control and examines viable alternatives.

Key Features:

- Reviews various scientific and regulatory aspects involved in the quality control of biologicals
- Provides an overview of the roles of various national and international regulatory bodies and accreditation agencies
- Presents advanced analytical methods, innovative technologies, and the integration of molecular diagnostics in quality control processes
- Explores the use of animal-based testing methods in quality control, as well as their alternatives
- Discusses guidelines and methodologies involved in the development of biological products

Overall, this book is an important reference source for various professionals in the pharmaceutical industry, including researchers, scientists, quality control personnel, and regulatory affairs professionals.

Quality Control and Regulatory Aspects for Biologicals

Regulations and Best Practices

Edited by

Dr Gauri Misra

National Institute of Biologicals, Ministry of Health and Family
Welfare, Government of India, A-32, Sector-62, Noida,
Uttar Pradesh, India

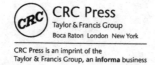

CRC Press
Taylor & Francis Group
Boca Raton London New York

CRC Press is an imprint of the
Taylor & Francis Group, an **informa** business

Design cover image: Shutterstock image number 142053856

First edition published 2024
by CRC Press
2385 NW Executive Center Drive, Suite 320, Boca Raton, FL 33431

and by CRC Press
4 Park Square, Milton Park, Abingdon, Oxon, OX14 4RN

CRC Press is an imprint of Taylor & Francis Group, LLC

© 2024 selection and editorial matter, Gauri Misra; individual chapters, the contributors

ISBN: 9781032697406 (hbk)
ISBN: 9781032697437 (pbk)
ISBN: 9781032697444 (ebk)

DOI: 10.1201/9781032697444

Typeset in Times
by Newgen Publishing UK

Dedicated to

The lotus feet of Shri Radha Krishna
and
Goverdhannathji

Contents

Figures

Tables

Foreword

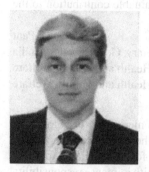

The importance of biological products in preventing, diagnosing, and treating diseases can hardly be overemphasized in the domain of biotechnology and modern medicine. The ever-growing advances in science and technology are continuously leading to overcoming various limitations. It becomes essential to maintain allegiance to ensure the efficacy, quality, and safety of these transformative biological products.

Quality Control and Regulatory Aspects for Biologicals: Regulations and Best Practices is a book representing a prominent and useful contribution to the field of biopharmaceuticals and healthcare regulation. The book would serve as a guide for professionals, researchers, regulatory authorities and students. It explores the varied world of biologicals diligently by delving into the basic principles of quality control, enclosing crucial facets like analytical techniques, manufacturing processes and product characterizations. This comprehensive book, edited by Dr. Gauri Misra, an expert in the realm of biopharmaceutical development and regulatory affairs, has paved the way for innovation so that patients all over the world get benefits from the latest advances in biological therapeutics.

In a time of rapidly emerging scientific discoveries and a transitional regulatory landscape, this book offers valuable insights into the requirements of quality assurance and provides its readers with the necessary tools to deliver high-quality biologicals to patients in need, consistently. The most remarkable feature of this work is the focus on regulatory considerations. There are regulatory agencies having a key role in protecting public health, but navigating the pathways can sometimes be intimidating. This book effectively addresses these intricacies, leading to the knowledge of accurate and latest frameworks of the global regulation governing biologicals.

As we move towards a future filled with innumerable possibilities in the field of biotechnology, this book will be a source of knowledge and inspiration to its readers. It ranges from pre-clinical development to post-approval commitments and illuminates the crucial steps and responsibilities that must be followed throughout the lifecycle of a biological product. It explores the interplay between cutting-edge science, quality control and regulatory aspects. In conclusion, this book is a noteworthy resource that empowers contributors in the biopharmaceutical industry to achieve their target of improving human health. It will certainly set a new standard in the field of biopharmaceuticals as it has covered various aspects of quality control practices and regulatory requirements. I applaud the authors for their perseverance in progressing the understanding of biologicals and their assurance in uplifting the quality standard and safety in healthcare.

As the readers embark on the illuminating voyage through the pages of this book, I am certain that they will gain valuable insight and the necessary expertise to make a positive impact in the dynamic world of biologicals. I extend my good wishes to Dr. Gauri Misra for her splendid work and valuable contribution to the understanding of biologicals.

Sudhansh Pant
Secretary, Government of India
Department of Health and Family Welfare
Ministry of Health and Family Welfare

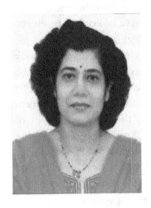

The advancements and emergence of biological products have shifted the healthcare scenario, promising new potentials for treating and refining patient health. This comes with immense responsibility to safeguard these biologicals in terms of safety, efficacy, and potency. This book, titled *Quality Control and Regulatory Aspects for Biologicals* comes with a comprehensive approach to make the audience aware of the current stringent regulatory practices across the globe to maintain non-negotiable high standards of biologicals.

The editor of this book, Dr. Gauri Misra is an eminent scientist contributing to the field of biologicals and research. She has used her expertise and skills to craft this comprehended view of biologicals. Each chapter of the book is particularly authored by scientists and scholars who have dedicated experience in the field of manufacturing, quality control, management, and regulation of biologicals respectively. Thus, providing a wealth of practical know-how to empower the readers to navigate the intricacies of regulatory guidelines and detailed quality control of biologicals.

The biological products' complexity mandates specific quality control processes from the stage of production to post-marketing surveillance. The book delves deep into the critical element of quality control including analytical methods, testing, and process validation addressing major challenges that arise during the stages of the process and also addressing strategies to overcome the difficulties.

The book also summarises the constantly evolving regulatory framework governing biological products that are required to keep pace with scientific advancements. Understanding compliance with this set of regulations is crucial for every stakeholder in the industry to ensure patient safety. This book takes a close look at the global regulatory outlook for biologicals, highlighting the specific requirements of the agencies.

I commend the editor Dr. Gauri Misra for her efforts and dedication in making the book, a competent resource. It will undoubtedly serve the audience's quest to know the existing regulatory norms in the field of biologicals. This book will be an essential addition to the libraries of professionals dealing with biologicals, fostering a deeper understanding of opportunities and challenges related to the quality control of biologicals.

Aradhana Patnaik, IAS
Joint Secretary, Government of India
Ministry of Health and Family Welfare

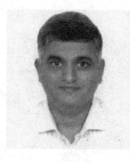

The field of biologicals has developed as a crucial pillar in the recent era of healthcare contributing to improved therapeutic outcomes and disease management. Advancements in the field of biotechnology and the growing demand for biological products put forth the importance of maintaining quality control and adherence to regulatory standards. It is with immense pleasure and anticipation that I introduce this comprehensive volume, *Quality Control and Regulatory Aspects for Biologicals* which explores critical aspects of the accelerating field of biologicals.

Dr. Gauri Misra, editor of this book, with her enormous expertise and experience in quality control, has amalgamated this book to provide consolidated and comprehensive knowledge about quality control in biologicals. She transcends the knowledge to researchers, regulatory bodies functional in different parts of the world, and industries to carry out quality production and management of biologicals. Biological products and in-vitro diagnostics have redefined medical practices providing novel and precise solutions to some of the most challenging health diseases. Nonetheless, this advancement brings high-end responsibility to ensure the efficacy, safety, and potency of novel biological products.

This book is a current necessity as there is a high demand for biological products and evolving regulatory insight to keep pace with scientific advancements. It is a cooperative effort by illustrious experts and scholars working in the field who have poured their knowledge, experience, and insights into this comprehensive guide. The book covers important topics, incorporating the development and manufacturing processes, analytical methods, and quality assurance measures specific to biological products. From the characterization of complex biologicals to the implementation of Good Manufacturing Practices (GMP) guidelines, every aspect of product safety and efficacy is explored by the editor. The authors also meticulously unravel the complex web of global regulatory requirements allowing readers to comprehend the challenges and opportunities in securing regulatory approvals for biologicals.

Dr. Gauri Misra is a senior scientist who is deeply committed to advancing scientific knowledge and fostering innovation. I am delighted to see this book serve as a guide for professionals invested in the future of biologicals. The insights and best practices presented here will undoubtedly inspire us to push the boundaries of scientific excellence and uphold the highest ethical standards in biological development.

Dr. Anup Anvikar, MBBS MD
Director, National Institute of Biologicals

Preface

In order to guarantee the safety, effectiveness, and quality of biological products, an intricate web of rules, best practices, and quality control procedures is required. The various chapters in this book investigate the varied realm of *Quality Control and Regulatory Aspects for Biologicals: Regulations and Best Practices*, and jointly shed light on the key elements of this important topic.

Starting out, Chapter 1, "Regulatory Aspects of Quality Control in Pharmaceuticals," establishes the scene by diving into the current condition of patient safety in India, in addition to examining the regulatory complexities of medicines. The chapter offers incisive recommendations to strengthen the legal and regulatory framework for drug quality and safety, demonstrating the book's dedication to promoting a setting with better pharmaceutical control.

In Chapter 2, "Importance of Quality Control in Biologicals," the importance of quality assurance and quality control for biological products is further explained. The need for strict quality control measures becomes clear as the effects of fake or subpar biologicals are explored.

Chapter 3, "Role and Importance of National and International Agencies in Quality Control Regulation," continues the story by illuminating the crucial functions that national and worldwide regulatory agencies play in the creation and distribution of biological products. This section emphasizes their crucial part in guaranteeing the distribution of safe and efficient medicinal substances around the world.

In Chapter 4, "Accreditations for Biologicals," the topic of accreditation is discussed in detail, including the crucial NABL certification (ISO 17025:2017) and the CDL/CMDTL notifications. This chapter focuses on the significance of using established standards to confirm the integrity and quality of biological products.

In Chapter 5, "Indian Industries and Biologicals," the amazing development of the Indian pharmaceutical and biological industries is highlighted. This revolution has addressed the accessibility of essential pharmaceuticals as well as established India as a trustworthy global supplier of generics. The chapter places special emphasis on the teamwork needed to maintain and improve this extraordinary trajectory.

With Chapter 6, the book delves even deeper into the world of quality control procedures by examining "Animal-Based Testing Methods and Their Alternatives in Quality Control Evaluation of Biologicals."

The next chapter, Chapter 7, explores "Good Manufacturing Practices in Quality Control," outlining the global relevance of GMP standards and highlighting how important they are to maintaining product quality.

The purpose of analytical methods is further explained in Chapter 8, "The Role of Analytical Methods in Quality Control of Biologicals and Stability Testing of

Biological Products," which goes into detail on the critical function of analytical methods in confirming the stability and quality of biological products.

Chapter 9 provides an in-depth analysis of two important regulatory organizations, the "Regulatory Bodies: European Medicines Agency (EMA) and Pharmaceutical Inspection Co-Operation Scheme (PIC/S)." The chapter describes their contributions to the pharmaceutical business in terms of quality assurance and safety, as well as their international collaborations and upcoming difficulties.

Finally, Chapter 10, "Quality Control Considerations Specific to the Development and Production of Gene and Cell Therapies," explores the cutting-edge field of cell and gene therapies while stressing both its distinct ethical and scientific facets.

These chapters were assembled to highlight the book's comprehensiveness with the aim of handholding various stakeholders, involving professionals, researchers, industry, and policymakers. Each chapter is a valuable resource because it is interspersed with advice from experts in the respective areas.

Acknowledgments

I am grateful for everything that has contributed to this sixth international book materializing.

Blessings from the Almighty and my parents, and support from friends and colleagues have driven this journey of conceptualizing this idea to see the dawn.

My deepest acknowledgment to my mother, Mrs. Kamla Misra. She continuously inspires me to give my best for the dissemination of knowledge. I am indebted to the divine blessings of spiritual guru, the late Bhaktivedanta Shri Narayan Swami Maharaj; my grandmother, the late Mrs. Shantidevi Misra; and my grandfather, the late Mr. Anand Swaroop Misra. I thank my principal, Sister Betty Teresa, who has been instrumental in making me believe in prayers, hard work, and my own capabilities.

My deep sense of appreciation goes to all the contributing authors who have dedicatedly given their best to make this book an asset. The support from publishing staff from Taylor and Francis has been tremendous. I pray and believe that this book will be a milestone in the field of Quality Control Regulation of Biologicals.

About the Editor

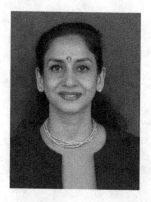

Dr Gauri Misra is working as a scientist and the Head of the Molecular Diagnostics and COVID-19 Kit Testing Laboratory at the National Institute of Biologicals (Ministry of Health and Family Welfare), Noida. She is significantly contributing towards quality control regulation of biologicals, ensuring the release of only quality biologicals in the Indian market, thus safeguarding public health and promoting access to good quality biological products and healthcare. She has extensive experience in the field of molecular diagnostics and cancer biology. She has completed her doctorate from the Central Drug Research Institute, Lucknow and postdoctoral studies at the CHUL Research Centre, Quebec. She is the recipient of many awards at different stages of her career. She has published more than 30 research articles in highly reputed, peer-reviewed journals, five international books, and six chapters. She has been invited as a speaker at various national and international institutes.

Contributors

Bhartendu
Syngene International Limited,
Bangalore, India

Brij Bhushan
National Institute of Biologicals,
Noida, UP, India

Tara Chand
National Institute of Biologicals,
Noida, UP, India

Khushboo Choudhury
National Institute of Biologicals,
Noida, UP, India

Ashwini Kumar Dubey
National Institute of Biologicals,
Noida, UP, India

Mahima Gupta
National Institute of Biologicals,
Noida, UP, India

Md. Arafat Islam
The ACME Laboratories Limited,
Dhaka, Bangladesh

Gaurav Pratap Singh Jadaun
Indian Pharmacopoeia Commission,
Ministry of Health and Family
Welfare, Govt. of India, UP, India

Manjula Kiran
National Institute of Biologicals,
Noida, UP, India

Anoop Kumar
National Institute of Biologicals,
Noida, UP, India

Ashrat Manzoor
National Institute of Biologicals,
Noida, UP, India

Gauri Misra
National Institute of Biologicals,
Noida, UP, India

Rashmi
National Institute of Biologicals,
Noida, UP, India
Academy of Scientific & Innovative
Research, Ghaziabad, India

Shruti Rastogi
Indian Pharmacopoeia Commission,
Ministry of Health and Family
Welfare, Govt. of India, UP,
India

Manika P Sharma
National Institute of Biologicals,
Noida, UP, India
Academy of Scientific &
Innovative Research,
Ghaziabad, India

Supriya Shukla
National Institute of Biologicals,
Noida, UP, India
Academy of Scientific & Innovative
Research, Ghaziabad, India

Priyanshi Singh
National Institute of Biologicals,
  Noida, UP, India

Satyajeet Singh
National Institute of Biologicals,
  Noida, UP, India

Shalini Tewari
National Institute of Biologicals,
  Noida, UP, India

Archana Upadhyay
National Institute of Biologicals,
  Noida, UP, India

1 Regulatory Aspects of Quality Control in Pharmaceuticals

Shruti Rastogi and Gaurav Pratap Singh Jadaun
Indian Pharmacopoeia Commission, Ministry of Health
and Family Welfare, Govt. of India, Sector-23, Raj Nagar,
Ghaziabad – 201002, UP, India

1.1 THE CONCEPT OF QUALITY: BACKGROUND

Globally, patient quality of life has been steadily improving since the turn of the century. This is mainly contributed to the advancements in medical technology. With the development of new drugs, vaccines and biotherapeutics, the healthcare industry has transformed, making the fatal ailments curable and, in some case, preventable [1]. It is crucial to comprehend "quality's" significance before entering and exploring it. But the major trouble lies in finding the exact meaning of "quality." Dr. Joseph M. Juran, who is regarded as the founder of key quality programs, describes "quality" as "fitness of purpose" while another author Mr. Philips Crosby, asserted that "quality is free," suggesting that any investment you make in quality will pay off. To complicate the thinking, some theorists say that quality has a different meaning to different customers based on their demand.

Maintaining the quality of pharmaceutical products is a top priority for regulators around the world in order to guarantee patient safety. The FDA's initiative to provide the Current Good Manufacturing Practices (cGMP) guide for the 21st century addresses the need for increased awareness regarding the significance of the quality of drugs [2]. The fundamental representation of this thinking is provided by numerous definitions that emphasize the ideal drug quality [3].

A high-quality medication needs to be both safe and effective. Consequently, it needs to be free from microbial contamination and should have a constant composition [4]. Healthcare professionals and consumers will then have confidence in the product as they are often not able to access the quality of the medicine independently. However, if a product's overall quality declines, it could have detrimental effects on the patient's health, which could be placed at risk by

DOI: 10.1201/9781032697444-1

a medicine quality issue, as well as the manufacturer's reputation, which could be tarnished among consumers and result in lower sales [5].

There are a number of definitions for "drug quality." The effectiveness and safety of a drug as stated on the label determine its quality for use. Additionally, it must demonstrate compliance with requirements for identification, purity, and qualities. If a product is of adequate quality, it must be designed to ensure that it will achieve its stated, desired, and intended purpose. And if it is not, the inherent flaw during manufacturing can also not be corrected. The quality of the drug depends upon the quality of the starting material, in-process controls and the knowledge related to packaging, labeling, and distribution [6]. The dynamic nature of pharmaceuticals and changes in color, consistency, weight, and chemical composition of the drug can be altered between production and consumption. Therefore, the effectiveness and safety of the active pharmaceutical ingredients (API), and finished formulation determine the quality of pharmaceuticals [7]. Thus, quality is inevitably taken to include safety and efficacy as depicted in Figure 1.1. Therefore, any defect in the quality of the product should be reported to the management and it is then their decision to investigate or to deny the release of the product to the market.

Testing the product, or "quality by testing," is not the only factor in determining quality. The manufacturing process to be technologically and economically viable, quality must be "baked" into every step of the design process. This is known as quality by design. In order to guarantee that the design enables the product to be replicated in routine large-scale manufacturing, quality is also based on "quality of manufacture." Current Good Manufacturing Practice (cGMP) regulations acknowledge the importance of manufacturing quality in the healthcare industry. In India, according to the Drugs and Cosmetics Act of 1940 and its implementing regulations, a drug is considered "adulterated" if it does not adhere to the cGMP criteria [8]. The pharmaceutical quality attributes are described in Figure 1.2.

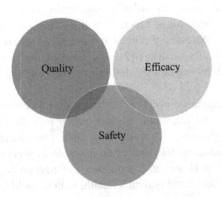

FIGURE 1.1   Relationship between quality, efficacy, and safety.

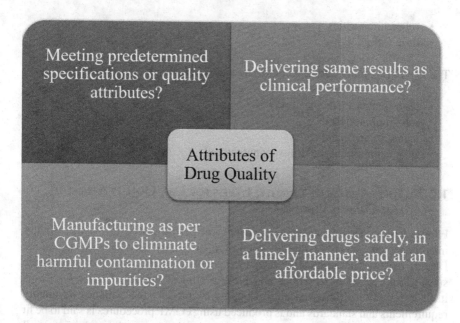

Meeting predetermined specifications or quality attributes?

Delivering same results as clinical performance?

Attributes of Drug Quality

Manufacturing as per CGMPs to eliminate harmful contamination or impurities?

Delivering drugs safely, in a timely manner, and at an affordable price?

FIGURE 1.2 Pharmaceutical quality attributes.

1.2 QUALITY CONTROL OF PHARMACEUTICALS

According to the International Organization for Standardization (ISO), to fulfill the requirements of quality, an operational technique known as quality control is used. ICH Q8(R2) (International Conference on Harmonization) defines drug quality as "the suitability of either a drug substance or drug product for its intended use. This phrase encompasses qualities like identity, strength and purity" [9]. With the use of quality control, the manufacturer is able to keep track of all the modifications made throughout development and production, providing quality assurance, enhancing public health, and even reducing the cost of pharmaceuticals.

1.2.1 AIM AND SCOPE OF QUALITY IN DRUG ANALYSIS

Pharmaceutical quality control testing plays a huge role in development and production of new pharmaceutical products. They also play a significant role in attaining quality assurance, enhancing public health through development of effective medications, and lowering pharmaceutical cost by exploring ways to reduce the cost associated with production and development of drugs.

Analytical investigation of the following substances is the goal of drug analysis:

- active pharmaceutical ingredient (raw material)
- intermediate products during synthesis
- products that could generate leads

- related impurities
- drug formulations

The aim of obtaining data can contribute to the following:

- high-quality medicine
- maximum efficacy
- safety of medicine
- high economy of the drugs manufactured

1.2.2 THREE ASPECTS OF QUALITY: FITNESS FOR USE, QUALITY ATTRIBUTES, AND CLINICAL PERFORMANCE

Fitness for use, quality attributes, and clinical performance are the three major interconnected aspects of quality, according to quality assurance or regulators. Despite the fact that clinical performance is not regularly evaluated, appropriate steps should be taken to reduce and prevent clinical failures. *Fitness for use* is itself a definition of pharmaceutical quality. A product that satisfies its quality requirements and standards and is produced using cGMP procedures is said to be fit for use. The limits on quality are chosen to ensure consistency in production of all batches. Understanding the connection between quality characteristics and clinical success is crucial. Because without this information, the limitations can be very wide, unnecessarily stringent or completely irrelevant to clinical performance. The worst-case scenario might also involve the identification, quantification or control of key crucial qualities. For the clinical performance, the established and defined quality attributes are adequate because they help in achieving tighter control on the variability level that could not be detected in patients without performing clinical studies [7].

1.2.3 COMPENDIAL AND NON-COMPENDIAL EVALUATION

Pharmacopoeia, a book of standards, provides the quality criteria necessary for a drug to achieve its predetermined quality features or regulatory specifications. The compendial assay is used in pharmacopoeias to assess the quality of pharmaceuticals. For evaluation of pharmaceutical products **compendial (pharmacopoeial)** or **non-compendial (non-pharmacopoeial)** methods are used. Pharmacopoeia are essential in defining testing procedures to assure the quality of drugs and are regarded as formal regulatory requirements in the event of a dispute. Pharmacopoeial procedures should be followed wherever possible. For products for which there are no pharmacopoeial method available, the justified manufacturer's standards that have been accepted by regulatory bodies may be applied [10].

The pharmacopoeias such as British Pharmacopoeia (BP), Chinese Pharmacopoeia (CP), European Pharmacopoeia (Ph. Eur.), Indian Pharmacopoeia (IP), International Pharmacopoeia, Japanese Pharmacopoeia (JP), United States Pharmacopoeia (USP), and other regional pharmacopoeias specify the limits of

API and pharmaceutical products to which a product must comply with. These specifications describe the essential quality parameters of the drug and are required for proper regulatory functioning [11,12]. The correct interpretation of a pharmacopoeial monograph, must be as per the current edition of the pharmacopoeia and in accordance with the general requirements and testing methods, texts or notices pertaining to it [13].

Pharmacopoeia provide specifications along with test procedures and acceptance criteria for pharmaceutical substances, finished pharmaceutical products and excipients. Throughout the course of its shelf life, a product should adhere to these requirements. Specifications are taken into account on the basis of the manufacturing process's quality attributes. Critical specifications need to be routinely validated. To ensure that the same quality is maintained at the end of the shelf life, the specifications are established for marketing authorization and these criteria are confirmed through batch release testing [14].

The quality specifications prescribed by pharmacopoeias comprise of tests that confirm the identity, purity, and strength of a drug and, when needed, its performance characteristics. The API and the finished formulations mentioned in the compendium have critical quality attributes divided mainly as follows: identification, tests for purity, and assays. The format for monographs in pharmacopoeias is as follows:

(a) **Monograph title**: it contains an international non-proprietary name (INN) approved by the World Health Organization and supplemented by the name of anion or cation (indicated as mono-, di-, tri-, etc.) and by degree of hydration. The drug substance monograph in the pharmacopoeia also contains the molecular formula, structure, physical form, and salt form.

(b) **Description**: physical properties of the drug, i.e., hygroscopicity, odor, and polymorphism state, if applicable.

(c) **Identification**: the identification tests should be able to identify the closely related compounds.

(d) **Tests**: this section includes (1) non-specific tests such as water, optical rotation, light absorption, sulphated ash, etc. (2) Impurities containing related substances and degradation products. (3) Impurities other than related substances, such as heavy metals, inorganic impurities, residual solvents, etc.

(e) Other tests such as loss on drying (LOD)/water, pyrogen test/bacterial endotoxin tests, if applicable.

(f) Purity tests with assay limits calculated on the anhydrous, dried, or solvent-free basis, as applicable. It determines the strength or content of the product.

1.2.4 PHARMACEUTICAL IMPURITIES

1.2.4.1 Definition and Types of Impurities

As defined by Indian Pharmacopoeia (IP), "impurity" is any component of a drug substance for pharmaceutical use or of a drug product that is not the chemical entity that defines the substance, or in the case of a drug product, not an excipient in the product [15]. The impurities in drug substance or drug product can arise due to manufacturing processes, degradation of substance or product, storage conditions, container, etc. There are three types of impurities listed in ICH Guidelines – Q3A: (1) organic impurities, (2) inorganic impurities, (3) residual impurities. Among the three types of impurities, the control of inorganic and residual impurities is easy. In drug substances, the toxicity of any toxic metal and solvent is limited and the limit of the toxicity is as per ICH or pharmacopoeia that guarantee that these cannot contribute to any side-effects. There are two types of impurities of drug substances – one is an API-related impurity generated by degradation of API itself (oxidation, dehydration, etc.) and another is the impurity that arises with interaction of API with excipients, container, reagents, or solvents. However, API-related impurities are generally mutageneic, genotoxic, carcinogenic due to their structural activity relationship.

The instability of drug substance and drug products is caused by a large number of excipients or residual contaminants found in excipients. Few examples to demonstrate the reaction of chemical entities with instability in drug substances are as follows: aldehydes in lactose, presence of reactive peroxides, benzaldehydes presence in benzyl alcohol, antioxidants in magnesium stearate, formaldehyde in starch and many more. Some specific functional groups in API that may be susceptible to degradation are oxidation, hydrolysis, and polymerization, etc. [16].

The potential contributors to side-effects are organic impurities of bulk drugs. Organic impurities such as starting materials, by-products, degradation products, intermediates, catalysts, reagents, and ligands arise from manufacturing processes and/or storage of the bulk [17]. As per ICHQ3A, the analytical procedures used should be validated and should be able to detect, identify, and quantify the impurities [17].

1.2.4.2   Need for Impurity Analysis

Nowadays, one of the highly regarded topics is the study of impurities in the field of pharmaceuticals. Not only challenging and time-consuming, but it is also essential to keep pace with the times. Impurity investigations have two main objectives, namely, (1) the regulatory requirements and (2) the scientific and technical requirements. From a regulatory perspective, impurities affect the quality of drug substance and drug product and ultimately affect the safety of patients. Major regulatory requirements to conduct impurity studies are the following: quality and safety of products; validation studies, i.e., specificity; determination of acceptance criteria; expiry date, retest date and shelf-life evaluation of product; study on stability and storage conditions and threshold limits' evaluation, i.e., permitted daily exposure (PDE), threshold of toxicological concern (TTC), etc.; the genotoxic impurities and degradation products that pose additional safety risks should be controlled in accordance with requirements of ICH M7 (R1), unless they are qualified for safety [18].

In addition to regulatory requirements, scientific and technical requirements also play a major role in impurity studies. Some of the important requirements are improvement of efficacy, formulation development and optimization, ADME and toxicological studies, optimization of synthetic and production processes, reference material manufacturing, stability improvements, and cost consideration of medicines [16].

1.3 REFERENCE STANDARDS

Pharmaceutical products are regulated during their entire lifecycle of development, production, storage, and distribution to meet various statutory requirements enforced by the drug regulatory agencies in a given setting [19]. Evaluating quality of pharmaceutical products during their lifecycle is an essential regulatory requirement for ensuring availability of quality medicines to the end-users. This is often accomplished by using official pharmacopoeia monograph methods and associated reference standards referred in the monograph. A reference standard is a highly purified compound that is well characterized and is used to calibrate and validate the analytical methods of the monograph [19]. The aim of using reference standards for pharmacopoeial testing is to achieve accuracy and reproducibility of the analytical methods. Therefore, quality of the reference standard is of prime importance as this in turn is used to certify the quality and efficacy of the pharmaceutical products.

Reference standards are used for qualitative (identification tests) and quantitative (e.g., assay and related substances) parameters to help ensure the identity, potency, quality, and purity of drug substances and drug products. They are also used for in-process monitoring, releasing the raw material, and during stability studies. The pharmacopoeial bodies or regional or national laboratories on behalf of regulatory authorities prepare and issue these reference standards. It is essential that the reference standards issued by the pharmacopoeia and their assigned values should be used for intended purposes and if used for any other purpose its suitability for new use should be demonstrated by the user.

1.3.1 PRIMARY VS. SECONDARY REFERENCE STANDARDS

Reference standards are broadly categorized as primary and secondary standards. Primary reference standards are compendial standards that can be obtained from pharmacopoeia bodies like British Pharmacopoeia (BP), Indian Pharmacopoeia (IP), European Pharmacopoeia (Ph. Eur.), United States Pharmacopoeia (USP), etc. In contrast, secondary reference standards are in-house standards established against the primary reference standards. ISO defines primary standards as the "Standard that is designated or widely acknowledged to having the highest metrological qualities and whose property value is accepted without reference to other standards of the same property or quantity, within a specified content" [19].

Secondary standards defined by ISO are the "Standard whose property value is assigned by comparison with a primary standard of the same property or quantity" and established by the users, contract manufacturers, and companies, such as chemical suppliers. Secondary standards are calibrated against primary standards for the specific tests by demonstrating identical characteristics to the primary standards. Secondary standards are usually used for routine quality analyses to determine the identity, purity, and assay value of the API in pharmaceutical formulation; however, in case of doubt or dispute, only the use of the "official" standard is authoritative. Stability of the secondary standard is established by recalibration against the primary standard.

1.3.2 ESTABLISHMENT OF REFERENCE STANDARDS

For the establishment of the reference standard, the pharmaceutical substance of a batch originating from the normal production process with acceptable purity (minimum 99.5% for quantitative standard) may be selected. Depending upon the use of the reference standard, the level of characterization is decided, e.g., for determination of potency, complete characterization, and qualification is required whereas for using the reference standard in resolution or identification only certain discriminating parameters are required. A reference standard proposed for qualitative analysis (such as identification) usually does not require high purity [19].

1.3.2.1 Reference Standard Material and Characterization

A reference standard can be broadly categorized as the following:

- Assays – used to estimate potency the active ingredient
- Related substances – to identify and quantitate degradation products
- Process impurities – used to identify and quantitate process-related impurities
- Resolution – used to establish system suitability during assay and impurity analyses

In order to definitely confirm the structure and identity of the standard, several analytical methods may be employed, including elemental analyses (i.e., C, H, N), crystallographic parameters, mass spectrometry, nuclear magnetic resonance (NMR) spectroscopy, analyses of functional group, infra-red spectroscopy and UV spectrophotometry. These methods ensure that the proposed substance is fully characterized. Similarly, the purity of the substance is determined by various analytical techniques and among them chromatographic technique for identification and quantification of impurities is useful. High-performance liquid chromatography (HPLC) is the most widely used chromatographic method in addition to thin-layer chromatography (TLC) and gas chromatography (GC). Other tests may include metal impurities [using inductively coupled plasma mass spectrometry (ICP-MS)], noncombustible impurities (i.e., residue on ignition), residual solvents [using gas chromatography (GC) with flame ionization detector], and water content (using a

Karl Fischer titrator). A collaborative interlaboratory study is usually carried out using different analytical methods to assign content to a reference standard, which gives the best estimate of the true value.

1.3.2.2 Storage and Stability

The reference standards are stored in containers to protect from air, moisture, and light to ensure that they are maintained throughout their shelf life. The name of the reference standard, content in the container, batch number, and name of the issuing body are given on their labels. Usually, the reference standards do not carry an expiry date and are considered valid for intended use until the batch is replaced or removed by the issuing body. Stability and integrity of the reference standards is monitored by a predefined retesting program using stability-indicating analytical methods to detect any significant change in their properties.

1.3.3 REFERENCE STANDARDS FOR BIOPHARMACEUTICALS

Biopharmaceuticals, as opposed to small molecules, have more complex structures that are not fully described. Biopharmaceuticals have a built-in batch-to-batch variability that is susceptible to changes in manufacturing. A well-characterized reference standard is essential to ensure consistency between different batches of the product and also to ensure the comparability of the product to be marketed with that used in clinical studies and innovator products. Quality determination and quality control for biopharmaceutical drugs often require the application of multiple analytical approaches, including physicochemical methods, assays that measure for potency, or a combination thereof. The characterization of reference standards for biopharmaceuticals should be performed with reliable state-of-the-art analytical methods [20].

1.3.4 PREPARATION OF SECONDARY STANDARDS

Secondary standards are usually prepared through interlaboratory collaborative study and pharmacopoeial methods are followed to assign the content by calibrating the candidate standard against the primary standard. The coordinating laboratory verifies that the candidate standard is as per the monograph requirements and dispatches the same to other participating laboratories along with the test protocol (with predefined acceptance criteria of the results) and result reporting form. After completion of the analysis, test results submitted by the participating laboratories are evaluated by the coordinating laboratory to statistically identify "outliers." Then the mean value is calculated by excluding the "outliers" and the same is assigned as the reference value of the secondary standard. A predefined retesting plan is also established to check the stability and suitability of the secondary standard.

1.3.5 REGULATORY CONSIDERATIONS

Regulatory authorities require detailed characterization of the reference standard while filing for a drug application to ensure that the product being tested against the reference standard has required content and its impurities (related substances and process-related impurities) are properly identified and quantitated. An insufficiently characterized reference standard is usually associated with delayed product approvals. It is also desired that the non-pharmacopoeial reference standards used should be of high purity and the analytical methods used to prepare them should be validated. As per ICH, analytical methods for quantitative determination of impurities must be validated to detect and quantitate the impurities [21].

1.4 PATIENT SAFETY

With growing complexities in the healthcare system and harm to patients due to healthcare setting, it becomes essential to monitor patient safety and drug safety. Both elements aim to deliver quality, effective, and safe health to the patients in an efficient and timely manner. The fundamental component of healthcare is patient safety. It has five major patient care elements: accessibility, acceptability, efficiency, effectiveness, and people-centeredness. Patient safety incorporates different aspects in healthcare settings that are crucial to delivering quality health services to patients. It covers safety regarding injection, blood, medication, medical device, organ, safe organ donation and transportation, biomedical waste management, prevention of healthcare-associated infection, and many more [22].

1.4.1 PATIENT SAFETY AND RELATIONSHIP WITH QUALITY

1.4.1.1 National Policies and Strategies
- India has largely fragmented regulations, laws, policies, and strategies on quality to be provided to the patients.
- The Consumer Protection Act, 2019 (CPA) address the issues of unfair practices, especially in private healthcare delivery systems but does not define the rights that patients have. These rights of the patients are mentioned in the Clinical Establishments (Registration and Regulation) Act, but this act is not implemented across the country.
- The regulatory authority of India, i.e., Drugs Controller General of India (DCGI), and price setting authority, i.e., National Pharmaceutical Pricing Authority (NPPA), ensures a check on medication and medical device prices to ensure that they are not overpriced.
- For implementing quality assurance programs in public health centers, the National Health System Resource Centre (NHSRC) is being designated as the coordinating center. Various standards are being prescribed by NHSRC to specify the need for quality and safety in public health facilities.

- To access the performance of a healthcare system, the Ministry of Health and Family Welfare (MoHFW) issues a nationwide report. However, this report focusses only on the quality of care with respect to reproductive, maternal, neonatal, and child health (RMNCH).
- Few private sector hospitals and independent institutions have implemented patient safety measures. But since they constitute a small proportion, their measures remain isolated and are not very effective.
- Accreditation of health facilities (laboratories, hospitals, and diagnostic facilities) through the National Accreditation Board for Hospitals and Healthcare Providers (NABH) is persistent. Public institutions are taking accreditation through the National Quality Assurance Standards (NQAS) developed by MoHFW. The International Society for Quality in Healthcare (ISQUA) is responsible for providing accreditation to NABH and NQAS.

1.4.1.2 Adverse Drug Reporting System and Surveillance Mechanisms

The mechanism for assessing the overall patient safety exists for various national programs like the Pharmacovigilance Program of India (PVPI), Adverse Events Following Immunization (AEFI), etc. The particular purpose of pharmacovigilance is to identify and report undesirable side-effects in compliance with the timelines and applicable regulatory requirements. As per ICH-E2E, the pharmacovigilance methods can be categorized as (1) passive surveillance (spontaneous reporting, stimulated reporting, intensified reporting, targeted spontaneous reporting); (2) active surveillance (sentinel sites, drug event monitoring, or registries); (3) comparative observational studies (cross-sectional study, case-control study, and cohort study); (4) targeted clinical investigations; (6) descriptive studies (natural history of disease, drug utilization study).

Good pharmacovigilance helps in identifying the risk and risk related factors in the shortest possible time, so that proper measures can be taken, and harm can be avoided or minimized. For certain events like pharmacovigilance, materiovigilance, hemovigilance, Adverse Events Following Immunization (AEFI) etc. the patient safety surveillance exists at national and subnational levels. But as this is voluntary reporting, all Institutes do not follow all the standards for reporting.

1.4.2 IMPROVING STRUCTURAL SYSTEM FOR QUALITY AND SAFETY

To ensure compliance with minimum safety standards, it is essential to develop efficient quality and safety structures and have an adequate quality accreditation and regulatory system. In India, there is a mixture of public and private health sector and also state governments have their own legislative, administrative, financing, and healthcare delivery models. Thus, a pan-India rational approach is required to efficiently implement the quality and safety measures of drugs.

Various ways to improve quality and safety structures in India are described below.

1.4.2.1 Institutionalizing Patient Safety

There is a need to institutionalize the existing policies and regulatory programs to make patient safety an integral part of the healthcare system. At national and state levels, measures should be taken for implementing a patient safety framework. Patient safety should be integrated in all vertical disease control programs, especially reporting AEFI in immunization programs, injection safety, etc.

1.4.2.2 Strengthening Quality Assurance System, Including an Accreditation System

To maintain the quality of drugs, it is essential to have proper a quality assurance and accreditation mechanism. It is essential that the central and state testing laboratories should be certified and accredited in accordance with the ISO/IEC standards.

1.4.2.3 To Establish a System of Reporting of Adverse Drug Reactions

- Sensitizing patients and healthcare professionals through seminars and conferences to report adverse drug reactions
- Strengthening the education system by incorporation of patient safety into the curriculum
- At national and state level, training courses and online or onsite training may be provided to healthcare personnel on patient safety

1.5 CONCLUSION

Patients lack the tools necessary to confirm the quality and safety of the medications made available to them, including their potency. A drug's journey from the lab to the patient is typically long and particular to each medicine. Enhancing drug quality, manufacturing, and marketing are crucial for guaranteeing patient safety and raising the standard of clinical research settings.

Understanding definitions and applying the quality requirements of manufacturing processes is one of the main challenges. Due to their concerns for both quality and safety, authorities must strictly adhere to the control of contaminants. There are few safety and efficacy data based on clinical trials available when a medicine is first introduced. This is mainly because clinical trials are performed in controlled conditions, and it is difficult to predict the side-effects and benefit-risk ratio under clinical settings.

Therefore, it becomes essential to maintain the quality of the pharmaceutical products that can be accomplished only by verifying these products using appropriate pharmacopoeia methods along with reference standards.

REFERENCES

1. Plianbangchang S. Public health and research: an overview. Journal of Health Research. 2021;35(4):374–8.
2. Haleem RM, Salem MY, Fatahallah FA, Abdelfattah LE. Quality in the pharmaceutical industry–A literature review. Saudi Pharmaceutical Journal [Internet]. 2015;23(5):463–9. Available from www.sciencedirect.com/science/article/pii/S1319016413001114
3. Lee DC, Webb ML. Pharmaceutical Analysis. Weinheim: Wiley-Blackwell; 2009.
4. Ozawa S, Higgins CR, Yemeke TT, Nwokike JI, Evans L, Hajjou M, et al. Importance of medicine quality in achieving universal health coverage. Plos One. 2020;15(7):e0232966.
5. Alshammari TM. Drug safety: the concept, inception and its importance in patients' health. Saudi Pharmaceutical Journal [Internet]. 2016;24(4):405–12. Available from www.ncbi.nlm.nih.gov/pmc/articles/PMC4908051/
6. Hejnaes KR, Ransohoff TC. Chemistry, manufacture and control. Biopharmaceutical Processing: Development, Design and Implementation of Manufacturing Processes. Elsevier Science. 2018;1105–36.
7. Woodcock J. The concept of pharmaceutical quality. American Pharmaceutical Review. 2004;7(6):10–5.
8. D&C Act. The Drugs and cosmetics act and rules; the Drugs and cosmetics act, 1940, as amended by the Drugs (amendment) act, 1955, the Drugs (amendment) act, 1960, the Drugs (amendment) act, 1962, and the Drugs and cosmetics (amendment) act, 1964, and the Drugs and cosmetics rules, 1945, thereunder, as corrected up to 26th May 1970. Delhi, Manager of Publications; 1971.
9. ICH Q8 R(2). International Conference on Harmonisation of Technical Requirements For Registration of Pharmaceuticals For Human Use ICH Harmonised Tripartite Guideline Pharmaceutical Development Q8(R2) [Internet]. 2009. Available from https://vnras.com/wp-content/uploads/2017/05/Q8R2_PHARMACEUTICAL-DEVELOPMENT.pdf
10. ICH Q6A. ICH Q6A specifications: test procedures and acceptance criteria for new drug substances products: chemical - European Medicines Agency [Internet]. European Medicines Agency. 2018. Available from www.ema.europa.eu/en/ich-q6a-specifications-test-procedures-acceptance-criteria-new-drug-substances-new-drug-products
11. Bari S, Kadam B, Jaiswal Y, Shirkhedkar A. Impurity profile: significance in active pharmaceutical ingredient. Eurasian Journal of Analytical Chemistry. 2007;2(1):32–53.
12. Keitel S. Inside EDQM: the role of the pharmacopeia in a globalized world. wwwp harmtechcom [Internet]. 2010;34(4). Available from www.pharmtech.com/view/ins ide-edqm-role-pharmacopeia-globalized-world
13. ICH Q7A. Office of Regulatory Affairs Guidance for Industry, Q7A Good Manufacturing Practice Guidance for Active Pharmaceutical Ingredients [Internet]. U.S. Food and Drug Administration. 2019. Available from www.fda.gov/regulat ory-information/search-fda-guidance-documents/guidance-industry-q7a-good-manufacturing-practice-guidance-active-pharmaceutical-ingredients
14. Uddin Md, Mamun A, Rashid M, Asaduzzaman Md. In-process and finished products quality control tests for pharmaceutical capsules according to pharmacopoeias. British Journal of Pharmaceutical Research. 2016;9(2):1–9.

15. Indian Pharmacopoeia. 5.5 Impurities. Indian Pharmacopoeia Commission. 9th ed. 2022.

16. Liu K-T, Chen C-H. Determination of impurities in pharmaceuticals: why and how? [Internet]. www.intechopen.com. IntechOpen; 2019. Available from www.intecho pen.com/chapters/65419

17. ICHQ3A (R2). ICH Q3A (R2) Impurities in new drug substances [Internet]. European Medicines Agency. 2018. Available from www.ema.europa.eu/en/ich-q3a-r2-impurities-new-drug-substances

18. Kelce WR. Drug substance and drug product impurities, Now what? MOJ Toxicology. 2017;3(1).

19. ICH TRS943 Annex 3. General guidelines for the establishment, maintenance and distribution of chemical reference substances [Internet]. 2007. Available from www.who.int/docs/default-source/medicines/norms-and-standards/guidelines/qual ity-control/trs943-annex3-establishmentmaintenance-distribution-chemica-refere nce-substances.pdf?sfvrsn=71064286_0

20. Berkowitz SA, Engen JR, Mazzeo JR, Jones GB. Analytical tools for characterizing biopharmaceuticals and the implications for biosimilars. Nature Reviews Drug Discovery. 2012;11(7):527–40.

21. Teasdale A, Elder DP, Nims RW, Wiley J. ICH Quality Guidelines: An Implementation Guide. Hoboken: John Wiley & Sons. 2018.

22. Janet Woodcock. Safety, efficacy, and quality remain top priorities as we continue our work to expand access to cost-saving generic drugs for the American public. FDA [Internet]. 2020; Available from www.fda.gov/news-events/fda-voices/safety-efficacy-and-quality-remain-top-priorities-we-continue-our-work-expand-access-cost-saving

2 Importance of Quality Control in Biologicals

Ashwini Kumar Dubey and Mahima Gupta
National Institute of Biologicals, Ministry of Health and
Family Welfare, Government of India, A-32, Sector-62,
Noida – 201309, India

2.1 BACKGROUND

In the last few decades, with the advancement in the field of bioengineering and molecular medicine, several biological products or biopharmaceuticals have been developed and marketed. These include various molecular, biochemical, and immunodiagnostic kits or reagents, recombinant products, enzymes, hormones, therapeutic monoclonal antibodies, various blood products, bacterial and viral vaccines, etc. [1–4]. These have become indispensable for the accurate diagnosis, treatment of hard-to-treat diseases, and prevention of infectious diseases. Therefore, these products must be marketed as a safe and effective way to diagnose, treat, and prevent diseases with consistent and predictable results [1]. The safety and efficacy of these products must be ensured at the production site, during packaging, and before release in the markets to end-users [2–5]. Quality control (QC) is highly valued in the biopharmaceuticals industry. The quality of their products is a crucial element and a producer's primary obligation. The production facility must meet any applicable national or international criteria for the product. The regulatory body of the nation of origin is also in charge of making sure that production site quality control procedures are followed [5–12]. Substandard or counterfeit medical products are a threat to public health, and therefore it is crucial to stop these poor-quality biological products from reaching end-users [13–18]. Quality assessment in drug testing laboratories ensures that the products are safe and exactly contained in the bottles or packages, as stated on the labels. By ensuring the quality, efficacy, and safety of drugs, biopharmaceuticals, and medical devices imported, manufactured, and distributed in the nation under the provisions of the Drugs & Cosmetics Act 1940 and Rules 1945 as amended from time to time, the national regulatory authority of India, viz., CDSCO (Central Drugs Standards Control Organization), in New Delhi, works to meet the national requirement [19, 20]. This chapter describes briefly the importance of QA and QC in biologicals and the consequences of counterfeit or substandard biologicals.

DOI: 10.1201/9781032697444-2

2.2   QUALITY ASSURANCE AND QUALITY CONTROL OF BIOLOGICALS

The term "quality" features a relative sense. According to ISO (International Organization for Standardization), "quality" is defined as *"the totality of features and characteristics of a product or service that bear on its ability to satisfy stated or implied needs"*. ISO further states that *"the quality of products and services includes not only their intended functions and performance but also their perceived value and benefit to the customer"* [21]. As per ISO, QC and quality assurance (QA) are parts of the quality management system (QMS). The QA includes all the systematic actions that are *"focused on providing confidence that quality requirements will be fulfilled,"* and the QC is the set of all the techniques and activities *"focused on fulfilling quality requirements"* [21]. Figure 2.1 depicts the QA, QC, and QMS as per ISO 9000:2015.

In contrast to chemical medications, the "biologicals" or "biologics" are typically obtained from viral, bacterial, fungal, animal, or plant sources by extraction, hybridoma, or recombinant DNA technologies [2-4] and are being used as biodiagnostics, biotherapeutics, and bioprophylactics, which are essential for the diagnosis, treatment, and prevention of many diseases. Most biopharmaceuticals or biologicals, such as monoclonal antibodies, conventional vaccines, recombinant proteins, and other biotechnological products, are being produced in animal cell culture. Therefore, unlike synthetic drugs and biologics obtained from microbial fermentation, these biologicals are more sensitive to various infectious agents, including mycoplasmas and viruses, which can cause diseases in animals and humans [2, 3]. Biologics or biopharmaceuticals are constantly at risk of various types of contamination, including microbial contamination. Vaccines, immune sera, antitoxins, antidotes, toxoids, blood and blood components, and other biological and allergy products are manufactured under strict quality control. An entire batch of biologicals can be destroyed by even a small bit of contamination. It causes a great loss both economically and healthily [3].

A poor quality or bogus diagnostic kit or reagents may result in an incorrect diagnosis of the disease owing to falsely negative results, which will ultimately

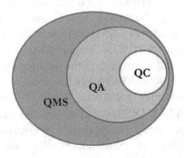

FIGURE 2.1   QA, QC, and QMS as per ISO 9000:2015.

result in a serious state of the sick condition. On the other hand, a physician can better control or treat the problem if they can accurately diagnose a disease using a standard reagent or diagnostic kit. Similarly to this, any subpar, fake, or adulterated biotherapeutic agent not only fails to work correctly on a disorder but also poses a major risk to one's health. If the bioprophylactics are of poor quality, they may also not act completely and cause negative effects on people. According to the World Health Organization, *"one in ten medical products in low- and middle-income nations are substandard or fake"* [14].

In June 2002, a diabetic patient in Agra, India, had paralysis shortly after receiving an injection of huminsulin (100 iu) from US company Eli Lilly & Co. Huminsulin is manufactured locally by M. J. Pharma in Halol, Gujarat, India, even though it is sold under the Eli Lilly brand. When the suspect samples were analysed at CDL, Kolkata, it was determined that they were "not of standard quality." A copy of the test report was forwarded to the national drug regulatory authority, i.e., CDSCO so that the remaining vials of Huminsulin in the market could be seized to save other patients [15].

The quality and safety of vaccines have a lot of significance as they are typically given to very many healthy individuals, primarily newborns, in enormous numbers as part of the national immunization programs. The manufacturing of vaccines is intricate, and there are not many suppliers to the global market. Governments or UN organizations typically purchase vaccines in large quantities through a supply chain with minimal middlemen. Although incidents are rare, this supply chain may be contaminated by subpar vaccines. About 60,000 Nigerian citizens received water injections in 1995 during a meningitis epidemic in place of the meningitis vaccine, which resulted in 3000 deaths [22]. More recently, over 100 infants in China died or became ill as a result of subpar hepatitis B and rabies immunizations [23]. It was reported that some 200,000 doses of faulty rabies vaccine were in circulation [24]. These immunizations offer no protection to the patient, similar to the fake meningitis vaccine used in Niger.

In India, about 150,000 vials of the oral polio vaccine produced by Bio-Med Pvt Ltd, Ghaziabad, in at least three batches were exposed to be contaminated with the type 2 strain of the polio virus in 2018. The children in the Indian states of Maharashtra, Telangana, and Uttar Pradesh had received these tainted vaccinations [17]. As per the CDC (Center for Disease Control and Diagnosis), the type 2 strain of the polio virus was eradicated worldwide [25], but its return within the community could have detrimental effects on health. However, due to India's widespread use of routine immunizations, the risk to youngsters was limited. The Indian regulator CDSCO found a few batches of the typhoid vaccine produced by Bio-Med Pvt Ltd, Ghaziabad, to be "not of standard quality" in early 2018 [26]. More recently, during the COVID-19 pandemic in 2021, several ampoules of counterfeit coronavirus vaccines were seized by Interpol in China & South Africa [27]. Such counterfeit vaccines cannot prevent the disease and thus contribute to its spread in the community [28].

Substandard, spurious, counterfeit, adulterated, or mislabeled drugs or biologics pose a serious threat to the public's health [14, 16, 29] and are estimated to cause

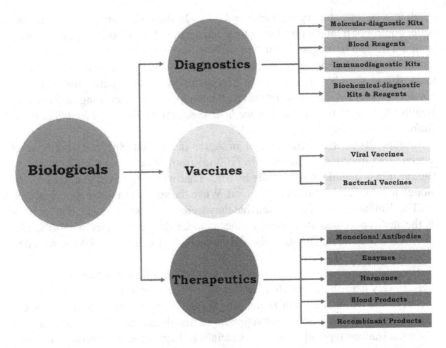

FIGURE 2.2   Different types of biologicals or biopharmaceuticals.

about 100,000 deaths every year globally [30]. Therefore, it is essential to weed out these poor-quality biological products or biopharmaceuticals from the hands of the end-users. It is necessary to ensure that the products are contained in the bottles according to their labels and also to ensure that there are variations from bottle to bottle and/or batch to batch. Laboratories involved in the quality assessment of biological products ensure access to standard quality biological products and biopharmaceuticals and thus safeguard public health by preventing the entry of shoddy, counterfeit, adulterated, or mislabeled products into the market. Thus, quality assessment laboratories are crucial in preventing consumers from receiving counterfeit or substandard medical products. The effectiveness of commercially accessible biopharmaceuticals, which are only licenced after careful onsite inspection and dossier reviews, should be cross-examined by more of these quality testing labs [5]. The biologicals are categorized as diagnostics, therapeutics, and prophylactics. Figure 2.2 shows different types of biologicals or biopharmaceuticals.

2.3 SUBSTANDARD, SPURIOUS, AND ADULTERATED BIOLOGICALS

Most countries and international organizations have their regulatory frameworks in place. To classify fake medical products, the WHO, FDA, CDC, and Indian regulator CDSCO employ various terminologies (Table 2.1) [14, 20, 32, 33]. According to the WHO, "substandard," often known as "out of specification," are those authorized medical items that do not fulfil their quality requirements, specifications, or both. The medical items that are not in compliance with national or regional regulations and laws and have not received examination and/or approval for the market in which they are advertised, distributed, or used are unregistered/unlicensed medical products. Falsified medical products are known to falsely advertise their origin, identity, or composition with malice aforethought [14].

The Indian Parliament amended the "Drugs and Cosmetics Act" in 2008, which is called "Drugs and Cosmetics (Amendment) Act 2008" [31]. This amendment has categorized the "NSQ (not of standard quality)" drugs into three categories, viz., category A, category B, and category C [20] (Table 2.1), which helps quality testing labs to characterize drugs.

Drug products that are spurious and adulterated are included in category A. The spurious medications disguise the true composition or brand of the product and the packaging for the medical product contains elements that resemble some well-known brands. These goods are typically produced by antisocial, unlicensed individuals, though occasionally by manufacturers who hold a licence. They may or may not include active substances. Drugs that contain adulterants, substituted products, or other filthy materials are referred to as adulterated products. Grossly substandard drugs are included in category B when they fail the dissolution or disintegration test, the active ingredient assay falls below 70% and 5% of the permitted limit for tablets or capsules made of thermolabile or thermostable products, respectively, or they fail to meet other quality standards and specifications. Parenteral preparations

TABLE 2.1
Regulatory Organizations and Their Terminologies to Categorize Counterfeit Drugs

Organization	Terminologies
WHO	Substandard/out of specification
	Unregistered/unlicensed
	Falsified
US-FDA	Counterfeit/fake
	Spurious
	Substandard
	Falsified
	Falsely labeled
CDC	Counterfeit or fake medicine
CDSCO	Category A: spurious and adultered drug products
	Category B: grossly substandard drugs
	Category C: minor defects

that fail sterility tests, endotoxin or pyrogen tests are too toxic or inappropriately poisonous, or contain fungus fall into this category of subpar products.

Products in category C have less severe flaws like emulsion cracking, formulation color changes, slight variations in the net content, spots or discolorations on the product, the presence of foreign objects, uneven coating, failure of the weight variation test, sedimentation in clear liquid preparations, and labeling mistakes [20].

2.4 QC TESTING

In a quality testing lab, the methods employed in quality testing are adapted from a pharmacopoeia, an international or national standard, or regulatory guidelines or procedures described in a research journal or developed and validated in the drug testing lab itself. Depending upon the type of biologicals various tests, viz., sterility, purity, potency, specificity, sensitivity, and precision and accuracy, etc., are performed to determine a biological product's quality.

2.4.1 STERILITY

Sterility testing is a crucial step in assessing the quality of biopharmaceuticals since they are constantly at risk of being contaminated by infectious microorganisms. The test sample is either transferred directly to the appropriate culture medium or filtered through a 0.45-micron pore-size membrane that traps microbes, after which the membrane is placed in the appropriate culture medium. Among various microbial culture media, soybean casein digest and fluid thioglycollate media (FTM) have been accepted universally. The inoculated soybean casein digest medium is incubated at 30–35°C and the FTM is incubated at 20–25 °C for at least 2 weeks to favor the proliferation of most fungi and bacteria, respectively. A biological product is considered sterile when a SAL (sterility assurance level) of less than 10^{-6}, i.e., one viable microbe per million sterilized products, is obtained [34, 35].

The biological testing for endotoxin, i.e., the lipopolysaccharide moieties of the outer membrane of gram-negative microbes, in test animals exerts many toxic effects, including a fever, which is the basis for the pyrogenicity test. As an alternative to this animal-based testing for endotoxins, the regulatory bodies have permitted the in vitro LAL (Limulus amebocyte lysate) assay, which is not only rapid but more economical and sensitive as well, and it requires a smaller volume of the test sample. In this assay, a small amount of test sample is mixed with the LAL, i.e., lysate of amebocytes from the *Limulus polyphemus*, which results in the coagulation of the lysate, also known as gelation [36, 37].

Mycoplasma contamination in biologicals derived from animal cell cultures can be detected either through the direct culture of the test sample, which allows for mycoplasma expansion in the broth as well as in the cell-free agar media with an observation of the typical "fried egg" colony on agar media or through indirect methods like fluorescence microscopy, in which the cells stained with the DNA-binding fluorochrome are examined under the fluorescence microscope [38].

On the cytoplasmic membrane, the stained mycoplasmas are visible as minute fluorescent dots. However, because this staining is not unique to mycoplasma, extra-nuclear fluorescence brought on by host cell nuclear fragmentation or bacterial contamination may be mistaken for mycoplasma. While the indirect method is faster and more economical, the direct method is more sensitive and time-consuming. Other indirect assays can identify mycoplasmas by analyzing their biochemical, genetic, and antigenic properties. It has been established that direct culture and DNA-binding fluorochrome tests are more sensitive than biochemical approaches. Ribosomal (r) RNA genomic sequences are frequently the focus of genetic assays for mycoplasma. Nevertheless, regulatory agencies must universally accept PCR techniques for mycoplasma detection.

2.4.2 PURITY

Biologicals or biopharmaceuticals may also contain low to high quantities of non-microbial contaminants, such as residual cellular DNA, peptides, proteins, media components, cell substrates, and reagents employed in manufacturing [39]. Biologicals made in cell culture from tumorigenic cell lines may also contain oncogenes that can transform normal patient cells. Because biologicals like cytokines, monoclonal antibodies, recombinant proteins, and hormones are regularly administered for longer periods and at higher doses than other biologics and conventional vaccines, the non-microbial impurities are expected to cause immunogenicity, toxicity, and reduced efficacy in these biologicals. Dot-blot hybridization, or qPCR, is used to quantify residual cellular DNA. Electrophoretic methods, such as sodium dodecyl-sulfate polyacrylamide gel electrophoresis (SDS-PAGE), and isoelectric focusing, and chromatographic procedures, such as ion exchange, size exclusion, and reverse phase high-performance liquid chromatography (RP-HPLC), are used to demonstrate the contamination of peptides or proteins. Sensitive immunoassays for antigens linked to media supplements (such as serum), host cell proteins, or reagents are also used to identify the protein contaminants [40]. The peptide mapping is used in demonstrating the variants resulting either from degradation due to proteolysis, denaturation, deamidation, oxidation, or due to mutation. The spectroscopic techniques, viz., NMR, IR, UV, and fluorescence spectroscopy, matrix assisted laser desorption ionization-time of flight (MALDI-TOF) mass spectrometry (MS) and MS/MS or tandem MS, are used in the characterization of peptides or proteins.

2.4.3 POTENCY

Potency testing is an essential component of quality control. Bioassays are a useful source of knowledge about the potency of biological products. This is crucial for assessing the consistency and stability of batches. At every stage of the biopharmaceuticals' development, from initial research to the final QC of the finished biologic products, bioassay data are essential. However, depending on the data needed and its intended application, bioassay types and designs may change. It is crucial to standardize using primary and secondary standards that have been accurately calibrated. Although in vitro treatments are frequently either unavailable or do not adequately address critical biologic characteristics of a product, in vivo bioassays are typically less dependable than in vitro techniques. It is necessary to verify bioassays for both the sorts of samples being measured and their intended use.

The specific amount of a biologically active ingredient required to elicit a biological response is called potency. Animal-based bioassays, cell cultures, and in vitro biochemical tests are used to determine the potency and efficacy of biologicals [41]. Because cell lines offer more predictable and controllable targets than primary cell cultures or animals, the majority of bioassays have moved on to cell lines at present. Results of bioassays are typically expressed in units of activity, which for highly purified biological products and reagents might be per unit mass of the specific biological component. The units of activity can be expressed either as per volume or as total protein for impure material [42].

2.4.4 SPECIFICITY

For diagnosing a sickness, a specific test is utilized since it rarely misclassifies individuals who do not have a disease as sick. A perfectly specific test ensures that no healthy people are mistaken for having a sickness. The specificity is the number of true negative outcomes compared to reference results. The specificity is calculated as follows:

$$Specificity = \frac{True\,Negatives}{\left(False\,Positives + True\,Negatives\right)}$$

A diagnostic test is considered very specific when it identifies all healthy people as negative for a particular disease. Conversely, another diagnostic test that incorrectly identifies at least 25% of healthy people with the disease would be considered less specific and have a higher false-positive rate [43, 44].

2.4.5 SENSITIVITY

Sensitivity is the number of true-positive outcomes compared to reference results. It is the percentage of positive samples that give a positive result in a test. The sensitivity is calculated as follows:

$$Sensitivity = \frac{True\,Positives}{\left(True\,Positives + False\,Negatives\right)}$$

A diagnostic test is considered very sensitive when it correctly identifies all (100%) positive samples whereas a test that detects less than 100% of the positive samples would be considered less sensitive because it misses positive results and gives a higher false-negative rate [43, 44].

2.4.6 PERFORMANCE EVALUATION OF IN VITRO DIAGNOSTIC MEDICAL DEVICES

For accurate insulin dose calculations and appropriate therapeutic decisions, blood glucose (BG) monitoring values obtained using equipment designed for self-testing by diabetic patients must be accurate [45–48]. Multiple self-monitoring of blood glucose (SMBG) assessments per day are advised for individuals on rigorous insulin regimens. Regular SMBG assessment is also advised for individuals receiving less intensive insulin therapy [49, 50].

Blood glucose monitoring systems (BGMS) are comprised of "glucometers and blood glucose test strips," which measure blood glucose (BG) levels in capillary blood. These medical devices are evaluated for their performance characteristics concerning their precision and accuracy parameters in a QC testing lab. As there are no statutory standards laid down in the Indian Pharmacopoeia or any other pharmacopoeia for testing medical devices in this category, the QC of such in vitro diagnostic medical devices is based on their performance evaluated as per the guidelines of ISO/IEC 15197:2013. As per the WHO guidelines for the BGMS precision criteria, the % coefficient of variation (CV) should be ≤7.1 [51]. As per ISO 15197:2013, the accuracy criteria specify that at least 95% of the results obtained with a BGMS have to be within ±15 mg/dL at BG concentrations <100 mg/dL and within ±15% at BG concentrations ≥100 mg/dL [52]. Those BGMS that comply with these specifications of ISO and WHO are considered "standard quality." However, the precision attained by experts does not always correspond to the accuracy attained by lay users, such as individuals with diabetes. Incorrect insulin dosing based on BGMS measurements can have a negative impact on glycemic control [53]. Therefore, manufacturers ought to offer high-quality BGMS systems that are user-friendly and error-proof.

2.5 CONSEQUENCES OF NSQ BIOLOGICALS

The accessibility of high-quality biologicals is crucial for consumer health. The distribution of fake and subpar (NSQ) biopharmaceuticals can have serious negative effects on both consumers and biopharmaceutical companies. The use of NSQ, hazardous, and ineffective biologicals or biopharmaceuticals not only imposes a serious threat to human health, which includes treatment failures, poisoning, disease aggravation, drug resistance, and occasionally even death, etc., but also has a negative impact on the branding, reliability, and profits of the biopharmaceutical industries. Additionally, it erodes trust in the medical system, medical personnel, and biopharmaceutical producers and distributors.

Quality control is necessary at every stage of the biopharmaceutical value chain due to the dynamic and complex nature of biologicals or biopharmaceuticals, as well as the cumulative impact of all production steps, from manufacture through packing and the circumstances of distribution, such as handling, transit, and storage. Therefore, efficient regulation of these procedures may substantially guarantee that consumers receive safe and high-quality medications. Increased biopharmaceutical trade globalization can result in the spread of hazardous, ineffective, substandard, and counterfeit medications on national and worldwide markets in the absence of effective regulation of biologics and biosimilars. India is regarded as the developing world's pharmacy; hence, there is seen to be a need for strong quality standards and enforcement in the country itself. To safeguard public health, the D&C Act, 1940, and Rules 1945, must be properly and effectively enforced to stop the sale, distribution, and consumption of counterfeit biologicals that are not of standard quality.

The inadequate QC at the manufacturing sites is the primary cause for the production of poor-quality or NSQ biologicals. The antisocial elements, through their deliberate fraudulent practices, also contribute to the production, sale, and distribution of such substandard biologicals.

2.6 FUTURE PERSPECTIVE OF REGULATION

It is crucial to regulate every potential future biologic because the "NSQ Biologicals" could have a detrimental effect on people's health as well as on the economy of the biologics businesses [2, 14]. In addition to the biosimilars that have been approved, there is a rising demand for a variety of biosimilars in developing nations, such as India, to address the rising number of off-patent medicines and monoclonal antibodies. Based on comparability about its quality, safety, and efficacy, a biosimilar product is similar to an already approved reference biologic. In India, biosimilars are regulated under the Drugs & Cosmetics Act, 1940, or any other relevant Acts as may be amended from time to time. DBT and CDSCO jointly created "Guidelines on Similar Biologics" in 2016, which describes the regulatory requirements for marketing authorization of biosimilars in India [54] for all stakeholders. QC laboratories are currently engaged in quality testing of approved biopharmaceuticals using validated protocols and are unlikely to significantly change their existing role. Numerous novel vaccines, monoclonal antibodies, biosimilars, and personalized or complex biological therapies are being introduced, and many more are in development around the world as a result of advancements in fields like hybridoma and rDNA technology, and gene and cell therapy. With these developments come new challenges in ensuring the quality of these biologicals to protect patients' health. To meet these challenges, the quality regulations and the business may need to evolve continuously. Patient safety and product quality are becoming increasingly critical as biologics become more complicated, precise, and personalized, and are used more frequently globally. Future developments will necessitate the creation of new quality laws with particular quality standards for viral safety, expression structures, product characterization, comparability, and other factors to handle the complexity of biologics. To incorporate industry best practices and cutting-edge technologies, regulatory guidance materials will continue to be amended and updated over time. High-performance liquid chromatography (HPLC), a common testing method, is used in several monographs. Compendial monographs have become obsolete as a result of businesses switching to ultra-high-pressure liquid chromatography (UHPLC) and other sophisticated technology. By the time the pharmacopoeias are updated to reflect the most recent technical developments, more advanced tools and methods have already been developed. The market appears to be evolving toward continuous monitoring, where outcomes related to the product's quality can be obtained in real-time. The current methods for updating policies, practices, and filings might not be able to keep up with the quick introduction of new technologies. Science has always advanced faster than standards of quality, so this is nothing new. It is more difficult for quality regulation to keep up with the technology's rapid advancement. By lowering manual errors and variability and enabling more rapid and efficient problem-solving, digitization and automation will also assure greater quality and compliance.

2.7 CASE STUDY: CHALLENGES AND LEARNINGS

In the year 2018, about 110,000 kids were administered with contaminated or adulterated polio drops in Agra, India [55]. One and a half million vials of three batches of oral polio vaccines (Batch Nos. B10318, B20318, and B010418) manufactured by Bio-Med Pvt. Ltd. in Ghaziabad, India, were discovered to be infected with the type 2 strain of polio virus, which has been eradicated globally. [25]. Maharashtra, Telangana, and Uttar Pradesh in India received the majority of these tainted vials [17]. The government, therefore, decreed that such contaminated vials should not be used since reintroducing the type 2 strain, which had been eradicated, may have major negative effects on public health. However, due to India's widespread use of routine immunizations, the risk to children was limited. Following this incident, around 46,000 doses of the OPV vaccine were seized, and the medical staff in Agra began administering injections of the inactivated polio vaccine (IPV) to stop the illness from spreading [55].

There are two types of polio vaccines: bivalent (for types 1 and 3) and trivalent (for types 1, 2, and 3). In 2016, the type 2 poliovirus-containing OPV was discontinued worldwide. Since that time, only viruses of types 1 and 3 remain in the OPV. There have been concerns raised about quality controls after it was discovered that the OPVs produced by Bio-Med Pvt. Ltd. in Ghaziabad, India, had the type 2 strain of the polio virus. Additionally, it was unclear how the aforementioned company acquired the type 2 virus for use in its vaccines. At the Central Research Institute in Kasauli, India the OPV samples were simply examined for their content's immunological effectiveness. As stated on the label, the Bio-Med OPV was tested for the immunological effectiveness of type 1 and 3 viruses but not type 2 viruses. Therefore, no one discovered that the vaccines contained a type 2 virus before it was given. This routine behavior needs to stop. All three poliovirus strains must be tested for in polio vaccines [56].

REFERENCES

1. Levi L, Walker GC, Pugsley LI. Quality control of pharmaceuticals. Canadian Medical Association Journal 1964;91(15):781–5.
2. Geigert J. Quality Assurance and Quality Control of Biopharmaceutical Products. Development and Manufacture of Protein Pharmaceuticals. New York: Kluwer Academic/Plenum Publishers; 2002. p. 361–404.
3. Shek WR. Quality control testing of biologics. In: Fox JG, Barthold SW, Davisson MT, Newcomer CE, Quimby FW, Smith AL editors, The Mouse in Biomedical Research. 2nd ed. Burlington, MA: Academic Press; 2007. p. 731–57.
4. Siddharth S, Nigam U, Gangwar P, Sood R. An overview of pharmaceutical and biological product quality Control Journal of Drug Delivery and Therapeutics. 2014;4(2):167–8.
5. Sargent EV, Flueckiger A, Barle EL, Luo W, Molnar LR, Sandhu R, et al. The regulatory framework for preventing cross-contamination of pharmaceutical products: history and considerations for the future. Regulatory Toxicology and Pharmacology. 2016;79:S3–S10.
6. Cussler K, Halder M, Hendriksen C. Future activities: ECVAM and the quality control of biologicals. ATLA 2002;30:225–6.
7. Halder M, Hendriksen C, Cussler K, Balls M. ECVAM's contributions to the implementation of the three Rs in the production and quality control of biologicals. ATLA 2002;30:93–108.
8. Halder M, Balls M, Hendriksen C, Cussler K. ECVAM's activities in promoting the three Rs in the quality control of biologicals. ATLA. 2004;32:93–8.
9. Mattia FD, Chapsal J-M, Descamps J, Halder M, Jarrett N, Kross I, et al. The consistency approach for quality control of vaccines - a strategy to improve quality control and implement 3Rs. Biologicals. 2011;39:59–65.
10. Shek WR, Smith AL, Pritchett-Corning KR. Microbiological Quality Control for Laboratory Rodents and Lagomorphs. Laboratory Animal Medicine. 3rd ed. 2015. p. 463–510.
11. Schutte K, Szczepanska A, Halder M, Cussler K, Sauer UG, Stirling C, et al. Modern science for better quality control of medicinal products "Towards global harmonization of 3Rs in biologicals": the report of an EPAA workshop. Biologicals. 2017;48:55–65.
12. Lüftner D, Lyman GH, Gonçalves J, Pivot X, Seo M. Biologic drug quality assurance to optimize HER2 + breast cancer treatment: insights from development of the trastuzumab biosimilar SB3. Targeted Oncology. 2020;15:467–75.
13. Nautiyal S. CDSCO-NIB survey of NSQ drugs to test 43000 collected samples in 10 govt labs. Available from http://pharmabiz.com/NewsDetails.aspx?aid= 89410&sid=1.

14. WHO. Substandard and falsified medical products: World Health Organization; [WHO Fact-sheets]. Available from www.who.int/news-room/fact-sheets/detail/substandard-and-falsified-medical-products.
15. Talwar P. India: Substandard Insulin being sold by US Company 2005. Available from http://lists.healthnet.org/archive/html/e-drug/2005-08/msg00073.html.
16. Johnston A, Holt DW. Substandard drugs: a potential crisis for public health. British Journal of Clinical Pharmacology. 2013;78(2):218–43.
17. Dey S. Contaminated vaccines put India's 'Polio free' status at risk. Times of India. 2018.
18. Tumbagi A, Balamuralidhara V, Narmada S, Mishra A. Not of standard quality drugs in India: a case study. Journal of Case Reports in Medical Science. 2021;7(3):11–6.
19. About CDSCO: CDSCO, New Delhi; n.d. Available from https://cdsco.gov.in/opencms/opencms/en/Home/.
20. CDSCO. Guidelines for taking action on samples of drugs declared spurious or not of standard quality in the light of enhanced penalties under the drugs and cosmetics (amendment) act, 2008 New Delhi: CDSCO, New Delhi; n.d. Available from https://cdsco.gov.in/opencms/export/sites/CDSCO_WEB/Pdf-documents/Consumer_Section_PDFs/DCC_Guidelines_Spurious_Drugs.pdf.
21. ISO. ISO 9000:2015 (E) Quality management systems - Fundamentals and vocabulary Geneva, Switzerland: International Organization for Standardization; 2015.
22. Cockburn R. Death by dilution: The American Prospect; 2005. Available from prospect.org/article/deathdilution.
23. Jia H, Carey K. Chinese vaccine developers gain WHO imprimatur. Nature Biotechnology. 2011;29(6):471–2.
24. The Associated Press. China rabies vaccine recall prompts changes: The Associated Press; 2010. Available from www.cbc.ca/news/science/china-rabies-vaccine-recall-prompts-changes-1.893814.
25. CDC. Polio Disease and Poliovirus. Available from www.cdc.gov/cpr/poliovirus containment/diseaseandvirus.htm.
26. Thomson Reuters. WHO plays down risk to Indian children from tainted polio vaccine Mumbai, India: Thomson Reuters. Available from www.reuters.com/article/us-india-health-polio-idUSKCN1MB3H1.
27. Davies P. Thousands of fake coronavirus vaccines seized in South Africa, China. Available from www.africanews.com/2021/03/03/thousands-of-fake-coronavirus-vaccines-seized-in-south-africa-china/.
28. Zaman MH, Sundaram R, Gabriel W. Fake, substandard vaccines and medicines spell trouble for controlling Covid-19. Available from www.statnews.com/2021/10/25/counterfeit-vaccines-medicines-spell-trouble-controlling-covid-19/.
29. Buckley GJ, Gostin LO. The Effects of Counterfeit and Substandard Drugs. Countering the Problem of Falsified and Substandard Drugs. Washington, DC: National Academic Press (US); 2013. p. 55–84.
30. Wechsler J. Campaign Mounts to CurbCounterfeit Drugs. BioPharm International. 2012:40–5.
31. Drugs and Cosmetics (Amendment) Act 2008, (Dec 5, 2008).
32. USFDA. Counterfeit medicine. Available from www.fda.gov/drugs/buying-using-medicine-safely/counterfeit-medicine.

33. CDC. Counterfeit Medicines. Available from wwwnc.cdc.gov/travel/page/counterf eit-medicine.

34. Woedtke Tv, Kramer A. The limits of sterility assurance GMS Krankenhhyg Interdiszip. 2008;3(3):Doc 19: 1–0.

35. WHO. Sterility Testing: World Health Organization. Available from www.who.int/ teams/health-product-policy-and-standards/standards-and-specifications/sterility-testing.

36. Iwanaga S. Biochemical principle of Limulus test for detecting bacterial endotoxins. Proceedings of Japan Academic Series B Physical Biological Sciences. 2007;83(4):110–9.

37. Levin J, Bang FB. The role of endotoxin in the extracellular coagulation of Limulus blood. Bulletin of the Johns Hopkins Hospital. 1964;115:265–74.

38. WHO. WHO Technical Series No. 872: Annex 3 - General Requirements for the Sterility of Biological Substances 1998. Available from https://cdn.who.int/media/ docs/default-source/biologicals/vaccine-standardization/who_trs_872_a3.pdf?sfv rsn=95b72196_3&download=true.

39. Federici MM. The quality control of biotechnology products. Biologicals. 1994;22(2):151–9.

40. Herman AC. Purity of biological products: related and unrelated impurities. . Developments in Biological Standardization. 1998;96:57–62.

41. Miles AA, Perry WLM. Biological potency and its relation to therapeutic efficacy. Bulletin of the World Health Organization. 1953;9(1):1–14.

42. Thorpe R, Wadhwa M, Mire-Sluis A. The use of bioassays for the characterisation and control of biological therapeutic products produced by biotechnology developments in biological standardization. 1997;91:79–88.

43. Shreffler J, Huecker MR. Diagnostic Testing Accuracy: Sensitivity, Specificity, Predictive Values and Likelihood Ratios. 2022.

44. Parikh R, Mathai A, Parikh S, Sekhar GC, Thomas R. Understanding and using sensitivity, specificity and predictive values. Indian Journal of Ophthalmology. 2008;56(1):45–5-.

45. Raine CH, Schrock LE, Edelman SV, Mudaliar SRD, Zhong W, Proud LJ, et al. Significant insulin dose errors may occur if blood glucose results are obtained from miscoded meters. Journal of Diabetes Science and Technology. 2007;1:205–10.

46. Breton MD, Kovatchev BP. Impact of blood glucose self-monitoring errors on glucose variability, risk for hypoglycemia, and average glucose control in type 1 diabetes: an in silico study. Journal of Diabetes Science and Technology. 2010;4:562–70.

47. Boyd JC, Bruns DE. Quality specifications for glucose meters: assessment by simulation modeling of errors in insulin dose. Clinical Chemistry 2001;47:209–14.

48. Virdi NS, Mahoney JJ. Importance of blood glucose meter and carbohydrate estimation accuracy. Journal of Diabetes Science and Technology. 2012;6:921–6.

49. ADA. Standards of medical care in diabetes—2017. Diabetes Care. 2017;40:1–135.

50. Elgart JF, Gonzalez L, Prestes M, Rucci E, Gagliardino J. Frequency of self-monitoring blood glucose and attainment of HbA1c target values. Acta Diabetologica. 2016;53:57–62.

51. Laboratory Diagnosis and Monitoring of Diabetes Mellitus [Internet]. IRIS-WHO. 2003.
52. ISO. ISO 15197:2013 In vitro diagnostic test systems — Requirements for blood-glucose monitoring systems for self-testing in managing diabetes mellitus. Geneva, Switzerland: International Organization for Standardization; 2013.
53. Freckmann G, Jendrike N, Baumstark A, Pleus S, Liebing C, Haug C. User performance evaluation of four blood glucose monitoring systems applying ISO 15197:2013 accuracy criteria and calculation of insulin dosing errors. Diabetes Therapy. 2018;9:683–97.
54. DBT-CDSCO. Guidelines on similar biologics: regulatory requirements for marketing authorization in India, 2016. New Delhi: DBT-CDSCO; 2016. p. 1–53.
55. Lavania D. Contaminated polio drops administered to 1.10 lakh kids in Agra District. Available from https://timesofindia.indiatimes.com/city/agra/contaminated-polio-drops-administered-to-1-10l-kids-in-agra-dist/articleshow/66102414.cms.
56. Basu S. After polio vaccine scare, questions on quality checks. Available from www.ndtv.com/india-news/after-polio-vaccine-scare-questions-on-quality-checks-1926802.

3 Role and Importance of National and International Agencies in Quality Control Regulation

Md. Arafat Islam
The ACME Laboratories Limited, Dhaka, Bangladesh

3.1 BACKGROUND

It is believed that the horse named Jim contributed to the creation of a law for biological product regulation [1]. In the year of 1901, children with diphtheria were treated with an antitoxin serum that was produced from the blood serum of horses [2]. The horse, Jim, delivered more than 30 quarts of antitoxin within 3 years, and then the horse was demolished due to tetanus infection. The serum from contaminated blood of Jim was accidentally applied to treat patients having diphtheria. This created the tragedy of the death of 13 children in St. Louis [1, 2]. The serum had been formulated in a local manufacturing system that did not maintain any established controls to confirm the potency and purity. Even there was no evidence of conducting inspections or quality testing activities of the terminal products. During the period of the St. Louis tragedy, a similar occurrence happened in Camden, New Jersey [3]. Nine smallpox-infected children died due to receiving vaccines contaminated with tetanus. Eventually, after the tragedy of St. Louis, Congress approved the Biologics Control Act in 1902 [4]. This Act gave the government its first regulatory authorization for regulating vaccine and antitoxin manufacture.

Under the 1902 Biological Control Act, the Hygienic Laboratory governed by Public Health and Marine Hospital service delivered rules imposing that manufacturers should be accredited each year for the production and market release of vaccines, antitoxin, and serum [5]. Industrial systems also were needed to undergo inspections, and licenses could be canceled if any violations found. Labels were needed to demonstrate the name and expiry date of the product with a competent scientist to control the production.

DOI: 10.1201/9781032697444-3

The Hygienic Laboratory issued certificates within a few years after imposing the 1902 Act to pharmaceuticals to produce vaccines for rabies, tetanus, diphtheria antitoxins, smallpox, and different serums to treat infection caused by bacteria, such as scarlet fever [3].

In the year of 1906, the "Pure Food and Drugs" Act was passed in Parliament, which banned the food and medicine items that were produced by mixing adulterated or inferior components or that carried false or ambiguous claims [6, 7]. However, this law did not provide a reference to biological products.

Another law named the "Federal Food, Drug and Cosmetic ACT" was passed in 1938, which was also known as the "FD&C ACT" [8, 9]. Under this law, biologicals were considered to be medicines or drugs. Although segments of the 1938 Act were functional for biological products, the Act did not update or obsolete the 1902 Biologicals Control Act. After the year of 1938, the proper supplies of the Acts of the year 1902 and 1938 were applied to regulate biologicals (Figure 3.1).

The Hygienic Laboratory was renamed to the National Institute of Health in 1930 [10,11] which became the NIH (National Institutes of Health) in 1948 [12]. As a part of the responsibilities, NIH contributed to control biological products until 1972, when it was moved to the FDA [1].

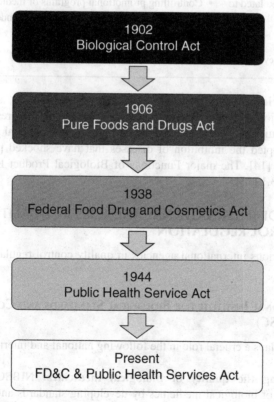

FIGURE 3.1 Rules to control biological products.

TABLE 3.1
Major Functions of Biological Product Regulators

Functions	Descriptions
License Controlling	• Control the license of the organization or industries involved in manufacture, distribution, import, export, and promotion of biological products
Assessment Program	• Perform assessment activities for the safety, efficacy, and quality of biological products and authorization after the proper assessment. • By assessing the safety of marketed biological products through analyses of contrary reaction reports.
Inspection and Surveillance Program	• The industries involved in the manufacture and distribution of biological products are undertaken for inspection and surveillance.
Monitoring the Quality of Medicines	• By taking control over the quality of marketed medicines.
Communication Related to Medicines	• Controlling promotional programs of medicines. • Circulation of information on medicine independently to professionals and the common people.

Source: WHO Policy Perspectives on Medicines no 7, 2003.

The Public Health Service Act, which was introduced in 1944, and the FD&C Act are the major laws that regulate biological products in the present day [13]. In the 20th century, the world observed great findings in biological aspects, many of which prompted the inhibition of diseases that have shocked populations in previous times [14]. The major Functions of Biological Product Regulators are listed in Table 3.1 [15].

3.2 ROLE OF INTERNATIONAL AGENCIES IN QUALITY CONTROL REGULATION

The role of various international agencies in quality control regulation are listed in Table 3.2.

3.2.1 NATIONAL INSTITUTE FOR BIOLOGICAL STANDARDS AND CONTROL (NIBSC)

This institute plays a crucial role in the following national and international fields:

(a) **Assuring the quality of biological medicines:** NIBSC assures the quality of biological medicines by developing standards and resources of references; testing to control the quality of the products and conducting applied research [16].

TABLE 3.2
Summary of the Major Roles and Duties of International Regulatory Agencies

Name of the Agency	Major Roles
NIBSC	• Assuring the quality of biological medicines • Providing systematic advice and knowledge to organizations • Ensuring the quality and efficacy of biologicals by control testing • Distributing international biological standards and reference materials • Carrying out an applied research program • Helping to introduce new medicinal products • Acting as a unique international interface
WHO	• Sponsoring countrywide medicine policies • Thorough strategies for standardizing biologicals
NRL	• Providing systematic and scientific support • Making laws • Providing support to maintain standards for routine testing services • Establishing a quality system in the laboratory
EQAAS	• Assessing the systematic functions of pharmaceutical quality control laboratories recognized by the WHO
NIH	• Maintaining the National Library of Medicines as the principal source of medicinal information in the USA • Conducting various general research centers
FDA	• Ensuring safety, effectiveness, and security of biological products through inspection programs. • Assisting in making the biological products more effective. • Controlling the criminal activities regarding the development of biological products
CDL	• Controlling the regulation of vaccines

(b) **Providing systematic advice and knowledge to organizations:** NIBSC is recognized worldwide for unconventionality, integrity, and scientific excellence. NIBSC provides scientific recommendations to a significant number of organizations, including biological medicine manufacturers, national regulatory agencies, the UK administration and European authorities, the WHO, and the UN bodies. Scientists of NIBSC contribute as members of vital decision-making authorities at both international and European levels. They also serve in the advancement of national and international rules that assist to confirm the safety and efficacy of biological medicines [16, 17].

(c) **Ensuring the quality and efficacy of biological medicines by control testing:** NIBSC works with UK regulatory bodies (e.g., Medicines and

Healthcare Products Regulatory Agency) and other European agencies to ensure the safety, efficacy, and quality of complex medicinal products. Biological medicines and vaccines are assessed and approved, self-sufficiently by the manufacturers, and distributed with a certificate prior to releasing them onto the market. Biological materials used in medication include bacterial and viral vaccines to treat diseases such as diphtheria, whooping-cough, influenza, rubella, meningitis, hepatitis, measles, mumps, and poliomyelitis. They also comprise medicinal products derived from human blood, such as clotting factors, immunoglobulins, monoclonal antibodies, hormones, cytokines, and growth factors.

(d) **Distributing international biological standards and reference materials:** NIBSC has a principal role in creating, evaluating, and distributing international biological standards and other biological reference materials. It is estimated that over 90% of these are supplied to WHO. The complex analyses used to confirm the potency of biologicals need the utilization of a typical biological activity – a batch of elements that have been allotted units of action and is utilized as a scale.

The effective application of vaccines, maximum biotech products in the treatment and several other biologicals rely on the readiness of international biological standards provided by NIBSC [16]. It also contains more than 2000 reagents brought by the CFAR (Centre for AIDS Reagents).

(e) **Carrying out applied research program:** NIBSC has internationally recognized researchers who conduct a global standard research program directly linked to its tactical objectives, supported by momentous external funding, and creating a remarkable publication output.

(f) **Helping to introduce new medicinal products:** NIBSC researchers contribute to ensuring the safety and efficacy of medicinal products through testing and evaluation facilities. They also assist to shorten the time required to bring new products into a clinical application by providing novel methods for their control testing.

(g) **Acting as unique international interface:** NIBSC plays a role as an international interface between product manufacturers, regulatory authorities, policymakers, and state-of-the-art academic research program.

3.2.2 World Health Organization (WHO)

The WHO is one of the main organizations of the United Nation that was constituted formally in 1948 [18]. The WHO has the following roles in regulations for biological quality control:

(a) **Sponsoring countrywide medicine policies:** the objective of the WHO's national medicine policies is to increase the utilization of affordable and high-quality medicines in each country. These strategies are important parts of universal health coverage of the WHO. This organization supports member countries to improve, implement, and control national medicines that confirm these medicinal products are properly prescribed and distributed, reasonably priced, and kept from spending high cost for consumers, and reachable to every part of states and regions, notably within health facilities. This method emphases on reasonable access to medicinal products through the progress of medicines to treat health problems that initially affect poor-income countries and originations based on recognized public health necessities. The WHO provides instructions on important medicines and health knowledge through policy manuals, technical meetings, and coordination with partners and member countries.

(b) **Through the strategies for standardizing biologicals:** the WHO arranges a biological standardization program in which internationally recognized experts participate to develop and revise the guidelines on biologicals. Through this program, the WHO exerts a role to prepare and establish worldwide biological references, written recommendations, and guidelines for these drug therapy products. The WHO circulates the biological standards in several ways, such as by creating a fast publication on the official website of the WHO and by arranging workshops to ensure the implementation of the guidelines or recommendations into regulatory bodies and manufacturers' exercises [19].

3.2.3 NATIONAL REFERENCE LABORATORY (NRL)

NRL takes part in the preparation of laboratory policies and coordinates in the activities of policy implementation [20, 21]. NRL directs laboratory functions among member countries and acclaim testing stocks, laboratory methods, and equipment [22]. NRL should confirm adherence to the approved standards (Figure 3.2). NRLs are selected by the related skilled authorities [20]. In regulating the quality of biological products, NRL has the following roles and duties:

(a) **By providing systematic and scientific support:** in order to ensure that the control of biological products is conducted efficiently and in a harmonized manner, NRLs provide necessary support to the concerned organizations [22].

(b) **By making laws:** NRLs set out laws to regulate the quality control of biological products [22].

(c) **By providing support to maintain standards for routine testing services:** NRL laboratories are high-quality laboratories, which are in charge of maintaining standards for routine testing in quality control laboratories of biological product manufacturer [20].

(d) **Other roles of NRL:** establishing a quality system in the laboratory, by approving the measurement system, by ensuring the traceability of the measurements at a country level, and by verifying reference materials to connections [23].

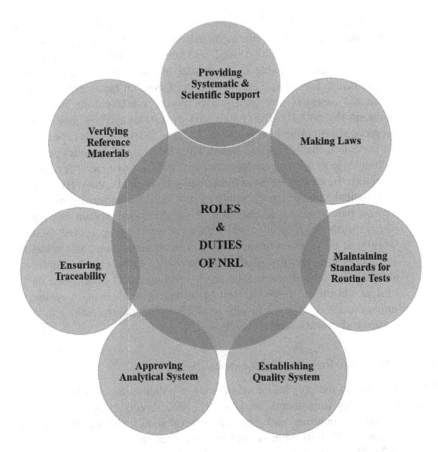

FIGURE 3.2   Roles and duties of the National Reference Laboratory.

3.2.4 External Quality Assurance Assessment Scheme (EQAAS)

It was founded in the year 2000 with the objective of maintaining the advancement of quality assurance in quality control laboratories of pharmaceutical industries in member countries of the World Health Organization. The WHO has planned and directed the EQAAS system in association with the European Directorate for the Quality of Medicines and Health Care. The motive of the EQAAS foundation is to assess the systematic functions of pharmaceutical quality control laboratories recognized by the WHO [24].

EQAAS provides each joining laboratory the chance to assess its activities through a private system of analyzing blind samples and to confirm its capability to accomplish a given analytical method within a web of national or local quality control laboratories [24]. This assessment can be defined as proficiency testing [25], which covers the complete testing activities of a laboratory, such as the reception and storage of samples, the analyses of the samples in the laboratory, data recording, the explanation of data, and making conclusions based on the data. The reports of the EQAAS study reflects the capability of the laboratory and the data of the reports cannot be modified unless approved by the WHO.

3.2.5 NATIONAL INSTITUTE OF HEALTH (NIH)

NIH is a part of the U.S. Department of Health and Human Services. The journey of NIH began from the year of 1887 when a one-room laboratory was made within the Marine Hospital Services (MHS) [10]. NIH is also known as the state's medical research agency, which contributes to important innovations regarding the betterment of health and safety of lives. NIH consists of 27 expert institutes that direct or support scientific works in several fields of health and diseases.

NIH is responsible for maintaining the National Library of Medicines, which is the principal source of medicinal information in the USA. The NIH also conducts various general research centers as well as the Division of Computer Research and Technology, which utilizes computer technologies to support medicinal research works throughout the country.

NIH has great contributions through significant discoveries to the improvement of public health and to saving lives. There are 171 noble laureates who worked at NIH or whose studies were funded by NIH. Some of the outstanding achievements are the development of MRI, explanation of the way for viral cancer, understanding of cholesterol control, and knowledge about "in what way a visual information is processed in human brain" [26].

3.2.6 FOOD AND DRUG ADMINISTRATION (FDA)

The FDA is responsible for saving people's health through programs that ensure the safety, effectiveness, and security of biological products and medical devices. The FDA also ensures the safety of the country's food supply, cosmetic products, and the products that discharge radiation [27].

The FDA is responsible for progressing public health by assisting to increase innovations that make biologicals more active, safer, and more inexpensive. The FDA ensures that people get the appropriate scientific information's that is needed to apply on biologicals to improve their health.

The FDA also plays a vital role in the country's criminal activities. The FDA accomplishes this responsibility through the development of medical products to respond to careful and logically evolving public health threats [27].

The FDA regulates the quality of biological products through the Center for Biologics Evaluation and Research (CBER), which belongs to the Department of Health and Human Services of the Government of the USA [28]. CBER conducts quality control activities by ensuring the safety, potency, purity, and effectiveness of biological products. CBER assists to get medications on the marketplace for recognized diseases and protects against threats of evolving infectious diseases.

The FDA has formed the Center for Drug Evaluation and Research (CDER), which monitors the medicinal products that are mentioned in the Food, Drug, and Cosmetic Act. The CDER assesses the applications for brand name, generic as well as over-the-counter medicines. This center manages the cGMP regulations of the US for manufacturing of pharmaceutical products. The CDER regulates which medicines require a medical prescription, monitors the publicity of approved medicines, and gathers and analyzes safety of the data about pharmaceutical products in the market [14].

The CDER receives significant public inspection, and thus applies processes that tend toward fairness and tend to isolate conclusions from being accredited to specific persons. The results on sanction will habitually make or break a small company's stock value, thus the CDER's decisions have a crucial impact on the pharmaceutical markets.

3.2.7 CENTRAL DRUG LABORATORY (CDL)

The CDL has an important role in ensuring the quality and reliability of vaccine manufacturing in the country. The CDL is situated at Kasauli in India, which is accredited by NABL and prequalified by the WHO. The CDL is the National Control Laboratory for assessing medicinal products, including vaccines and antisera. The lab has the command of National Regulations of Vaccines formulated indigenously for the national market, immunization program of the government of India, export, and for those imported to the country.

The CDL has been founded under the rules of the Drugs & Cosmetic ACT 1940. Documentation system of CDL is based on the standards of ISO/IEC 17025:2005. The CDL receives about 7000 immunobiological batches in each year in order to testing or prerelease certification [29].

The WHO has authorized the CDL to distribute local working reference standards for the pertussis vaccine. The CDL also provides various other National Reference Standards of different vaccines to all the vaccine producers in India. The available reference standards have been given below:

(a) Diphtheria Antitoxin (In Vivo and In Vitro)
(b) Tetanus Antitoxin (In Vivo and In Vitro)
(c) Diphtheria Toxoid (G. pig Challenge method)
(d) Tetanus Toxoid (G. pig Challenge method)
(e) Pertussis Vaccine (RWRS)
(f) Bacillus-Calmette-Guerin Vaccine
(g) Anti Rabies serum
(h) Snake venom (Cobra, Krait, Rusell Viper and Saw Scaled Viper)
(i) Rabies Vaccine
(j) Measles Vaccine
(k) Mumps Vaccine
(l) Rubella Vaccine

(m) Poliomyelitis Vaccine (bivalent OPV 1 +3)
(n) Poliomyelitis Vaccine (m OPV Type I)
(o) Poliomyelitis Vaccine (m OPV Type III)

3.3 ROLE OF NATIONAL AGENCIES IN QUALITY CONTROL REGULATION

The role of various national agencies in quality control regulation are listed in Table 3.3.

3.3.1 CENTRAL DRUGS STANDARD CONTROL ORGANIZATION (CDSCO)

The CDSCO's headquarter is situated at FDA Bhawan, New Delhi. It has six regional offices, four subregional offices, and 13 port offices. It also has seven laboratories all over the country. The CDSCO is India's national regulatory agency, which works for cosmetics, biological products, and medical devices. It has identical functions to EMA (European Medicines Agency, Amsterdam); PMDA (Pharmaceuticals and Medical Devices Agency, Japan), the FDA (Food and Drug Administration, United States); the MHRA (Medicines and Healthcare Products Regulatory Agency, UK), and NMPA (National Medical Products Administration, China). The government of India has planned to review all medical devices, including contraceptives and implants, within the CDSCO [30].

TABLE 3.3
Summary of the Major Roles and Duties of National Regulatory Agencies

Name of the Agency	Major Roles
CDSCO	• Approving new drugs • Conducting clinical trials of new drugs • Maintaining quality standards of imported biologicals
IPC	• Regularly updating the standards of medicines commonly used in the country • Publishing papers about the progress in quality of medicines • Updating guidelines of Indian Pharmacopoeia
CRI	• Formulation of vaccine • Development of human resources • Serving as a referral center for diseases in the country
NIB	• Monitoring the quality of biologicals that are formulated and imported in the country • Implementation of the Indian Hemovigilance Programme to provide secure blood transfusion practices • Preparation of National Reference Standards/Sera Panels

The CDSCO is responsible for recognizing new drugs, conducting clinical trials through the country, establishing the standards for medicinal products, and maintaining the quality of imported medicines [31]. This organization conducts its function under the supervision of National Pharmacovigilance Advisory Committee [32, 33].

The CDSCO is continually progressing to establish transparency, liability, and consistency in its regular services in order to ensure safety, efficacy, and quality of the biological products manufactured, traded in, and distributed in the country [31].

The CDSCO works under the Directorate General of Health Services and it has the following functions:

(a) Approving new biological products and conducting clinical trials.
(b) Providing registration and license for importing.
(c) Approving license for blood banks, large volume parenteral products (LVP), r-DNA products, vaccines, and several medical devices.
(d) Revision of D&C Act and Rules.
(e) If necessary, outlawing of drugs and cosmetics.
(f) Allowance of test license, individual license, NOCs for products to be exported.
(g) Testing new biological products.
(h) Oversight and market investigation through inspectorate of the center in addition to the government authority.

3.3.2 INDIAN PHARMACOPOEIA COMMISSION (IPC)

The IPC is a self-directed institute controlled by the Indian Government's Ministry of Health and Family Welfare. The IPC is created to establish standards of medicines, in the country. Its basic role is to update the standards of medicines commonly needed for treating diseases that are predominant in this country regularly. It publishes official papers for the advancement of the quality of medicines by adding new and updating existing guidelines in the system of Indian Pharmacopoeia [34]. IP recommends standards for distinctiveness, cleanliness, and strength of medicines required for treating diseases of humans and animals [35].

IPC plays the following roles to regulate biological products:

(a) **By publishing Indian Pharmacopoeia (IP):** IPC publish Indian Pharmacopoeia (IP) and the Indian Government support IPC to publish IP. Indian Pharmacopoeia is known as the legally imposable book of standards for the pharmaceutical products being produced or sold in India [34]. The objective of IP is to assist in obtaining a license of manufacturing, inspection, and supply of pharmaceutical products. IPC publish IP regularly as a significant command to improve health by confirming the quality, safety, and efficacy of pharmaceutical products [36].

(b) **By publishing National Formulary of India (NFI):** IPC publish National Formulary of India (NFI) on behalf of the Health Ministry of the Indian Government. IPC got this accountability since the year of 2008 [37, 38]. A formulary is a guide containing information related to pharmaceutical products. The formulary may contain legislative and governing information relating to the recommending and supplying of pharmaceutical products.

NFI mainly focuses on accessible and reasonable drugs that are applicable to the medication of diseases in India. NFI has been implemented from the WHO Typical Formulary and systematically updated for its content, particularly keeping in view the consumer in India [37].

When medicinal products are selected to be included in the NFI, then various attributes are considered for the selection, such as the positive and negative effects of the product/s, the range of their application in recent practice, and their accessibility in India. Therefore, the NFI signifies a wide consent of medical judgment in the case of medicinal products and their preparations and delivers medical professionals with cautiously particular healing agents of verified effectiveness, which build the foundation of national medicine treatment [39].

(c) **By issuing reference standards:** IPC has the accountability to issue reference substances and standard formulations of antibiotics. IP reference substances are denoted as IPRS. These are used in respect of arbitration and standardizing the working standards at consistent intervals. IPRS are standardized against the global standards and reference formulations recognized by the WHO [40].

(d) **By the Research and Development Division:** IPC has the mission and vision to bring out the highest standards of pharmaceutical products through its analytical research and development (AR&D) division. The AR&D division of IPC regularly circulates the variations to analytical test procedures consistent with state-of-the-art technological demands. Through the AR&D division, the IPC validates and verifies the monographs that are included in the IP [41].

(e) **By maintaining quality management system:** the IPC has a Quality Assurance Department (QA) through which it controls the quality management system. The QA Department plays an important role in controlling the quality standards of pharmaceutical product manufacturing [42].

3.3.3 CENTRAL RESEARCH INSTITUTE (CRI)

The CRI is an innovator in the field of vaccines in India as well as in the world. CRI was established in the year of 1905 with the purpose of conducting scientific works in the field of medicines and public health, formulation of vaccines and antisera, development of human resources and to serve as a referral center of the country for diseases. This institute works with the vision to produce vaccines against evolving diseases by maintaining cGMP compliance and to develop as a training hub in respect of immunobiologicals.

The organization has achieved various milestones over the period of its journey of 117 years. During this time the CRI has been endlessly contributing to Health Program of the Country. The objective of the organization is to manufacture lifesaving medicines, quality monitoring activities, educating and training the microbiological and vaccinilogical aspects [43].

CRI is the first Central Government Institute to have cGMP compliant setup for vaccine manufacturing. This institute played an outstanding role in vaccine manufacturing at the time of the Second World War for the vaccination of troops to retain them fit for fighting.

3.3.4 National Institute of Biologicals (NIB)

The NIB is one of the major self-directed organizations of India's Ministry of Health and Family welfare that is involved in regulating quality of the biologicals that are formulated and imported in India. The NIB was established in 1992, and is located in Noida, Uttar Pradesh [44].

To achieve the national obligation for ensuring the quality of biologicals to protect human health, NIB has the following attempts:

(a) **Fulfilment of the requirements of international standards:** the NIB is devoted to fulfil the requirements of ISO/IEC 17025:2017 to approve accurate and dependable results through unbiased and constant operation and upholding confidentiality.

(b) **Improvement of the quality management system:** NIB has established methods and actions to review the quality objectives in a routine manner, thus continually improving the efficiency of the quality management system [45].

(c) **Quality control of biologicals used in a broad range of treatment:** the NIB is conducting quality control programs for biologicals that are used for a wide range of treatments, such as insulin, blood products, erythropoietin, analytical kits (e.g., HIV, HBV, HCV), and therapeutic monoclonal antibodies used to cure cancer diseases. NIB conducts the quality control program by following the Drugs & Cosmetics Act and Rules 1945. Furthermore, the institute is involved in preparation of national reference standards, and sera panels [45].

(d) **Quality control program together with the WHO:** the NIB conducts quality control works in collaboration with WHO for immunodiagnostic kits of HBsAg, HCV, HIV, and syphilis. The institute also helps in in vitro diagnostics that are aimed for the WHO prequalification program [44].

(e) **Contribution as a Central Laboratory:** the NIB act as the Central Drugs Laboratory and Central Testing Laboratory for Medical Device under the legal requirements of ISO/IEC 17025:2017. The biologicals are tested by following the approved standards as mentioned in Indian Pharmacopoeia or International Guidelines [45].

(f) **Testing biologicals involving government-recognized scientists:** some of the NIB scientists are recognized as Government Analysts who perform tests for biologicals as per legal standards [45]. The scientists of NIB are dedicated towards their work by following the orders and roles precisely. Some of the functions have been given below:

- to confirm the quality of biologicals that are traded in and produced in the Indian market;
- to work on the finalization of the specifications for pharmaceutical products to be included in Indian Pharmacopoeia;
- to create National Reference Standards for biologicals;
- to build up technical individuals by training them about the quality control of biologicals;
- to work with other countrywide and worldwide scientific organizations/ institutions in improving technologies;
- to keep up-to-date scientific progresses made concerning with quality assessment of biologicals;
- to cover procedural knowledge at the time of joint investigations of the manufacturing area of biologicals with the personnel of CDSCO;
- to implement the Indian Hemovigilance Programme to provide secure blood transfusion practices.

(g) **Proper Laboratory Facility:** the NIB is facilitated with a Laboratory and Animal Facility, which was built in 2006. There are biosafety level-2 laboratories developed with state-of-the-art scientific equipment for conducting test of biologicals [44].

3.4 CONCLUSION

The overall purpose of the quality regulation of biological products is to ensure the safety of human beings and animals. A safe medicine is one that has low risks to the patient, the extent of the benefit predictable, and the substitutes available. The choice to use a biological product involves balancing the benefits to be gained with the potential risks. Regulatory agencies around the world are playing a vital role to fulfill these challenges. Since the discovery of the medication system, several regulatory acts had been implemented considering the proper application of the medication against health problems. With the continual emergence of health issues, the formulation of biological products will be continued. If the formulation and distribution of these biological products are properly maintained by following the existing rules and regulations of local and international authorities, there will be fewer complications in health issues. Thus, it will help in the development of a healthy and stable world in the upcoming days.

REFERENCES

1. Bren L. The road to the biotech revolution: highlights of 100 years of biologics regulation. FDA Consumer 2006;40(1):50–7. PMID: 16528828.
2. DeHovitz RE. The 1901 St Louis incident: the first modern medical disaster. Pediatrics. 2014;133(6):964–5. doi:10.1542/peds.2013-2817. PMID: 24864186.
3. Hutt PB. The evolution of federal regulation of human drugs in the united states: an historical essay. American Journal of Law and Medicine. 2018;44(2-3):403–451. doi:10.1177/0098858818789421. PMID: 30106657.
4. McWilliams DE. Reforming drug approval in the United States: measures necessary to alleviate the cash crunch faced by small. Third Year Paper: Harvard Law School. 1995.
5. Lilienfeld DE. The first pharmacoepidemiologic investigations: national drug safety policy in the United States, 1901-1902. Perspectives in Biology and Medicine [Internet]. 2008; 51:188–98. Available from www.semanticscholar.org/paper/The-First-Pharmacoepidemiologic-Investigations%3A-in-Lilienfeld/df0d7e0793594 f0e66f3c0401d113b2d65e8de97
6. U.S. Food and Drug Administration. The history of drug regulation [Internet]. U.S.: United State Government; 2018. Available from www.fda.gov/about-fda/fda-history/history-drug-regulation
7. Osakwe O, Rizvi AS, Pharmaceutical regulation: social aspects of drug discovery, development and commercialization [Internet]. Edition. Saint Louis: Elsevier Science; 2016. Available from www.sciencedirect.com/book/9780128022207/soc ial-aspects-of-drug-discovery-development-and-commercialization.   doi:10.1016/ C2014-0-02679-2
8. Meadows M. Promoting safe & effective drugs for 100 years [internet]. FDA Consumer Magazine: U.S. Food and Drug Administration; 2006. 8 p. Report No. Available from www.fda.gov/media/110482/download
9. Lee PR, Herzstein J. International drug regulation. Annual Review of Public Health. 1986;7:217–35. doi:10.1146/annurev.pu.07.050186.001245. PMID: 3521644.
10. National Institutes of Health. A short history of national institutes of health [Internet]. Bethesda, MD. Department of Health and Human Services. Available from https://history.nih.gov/display/history/WWI+and+the+Ransdell+Act+of+1930
11. Murray DM. Prevention research at the National Institutes of Health. Public Health Report. 2017;132(5):535–38. doi:10.1177/0033354917720943. PMID: 28809604; PMCID: PMC5593237.
12. Crocoll S. NIH in history-the centennial anchor: a symbol of NIH's maritime origins [Internet]. NIH Intramural Research Program; 2014. 13 p. Report No. 22(2). Available from https://irp.nih.gov/system/files/media/file/2022-01/catalyst_v22i2-CLR_0.pdf
13. Public Health Service Act, 1944. Public Health Report. 1994;109(4):468. PMID: 8041843; PMCID: PMC1403520.
14. Wikipedia Contributors. Center for Drug Evaluation and Research [Internet]. Wikipedia. Available from https://en.wikipedia.org/w/index.php?title=Center_for_Drug_Evaluation_and_Research&oldid=1129205610

15. World Health Organization. Effective medicines regulation: ensuring safety, efficacy and quality [Internet]. 2003. 6 p. Report No.: WHO/EDM/2003.2. Available from https://apps.who.int/iris/handle/10665/68391

16. National Institute for Biological Standards and Control (NIBSC). About us [Internet]. Medicines & Healthcare Products Regulatory Agency. 2022. Available from www.nibsc.org/about_us.aspx

17. Wikipedia contributors. National Institute for Biological Standards and Control [Internet]. Wikipedia. 2022. Available from https://en.wikipedia.org/wiki/National_Institute_for_Biological_Standards_and_Control#History

18. Pardeshi AA. Role and function of drug regulatory authorities in the backdrop of good governance [dissertation on the Internet]. SSRN 1748629. 2011. 2022. Available from https://papers.ssrn.com/sol3/papers.cfm?abstract_id=1748629

19. World Health Organization (WHO). Promoting national medicines policies [Internet]. 2022. Available from www.who.int/activities/promoting-national-medicines-policies.

20. Southern African Development Community (SADC). Functions and Minimum Standards for National Reference Laboratories in the SADC Region [Internet]. Botswana: Directorate of Social and Human Development and Special Programs; 2009. 25 p. Available from https://dev-www.sadc.int/files/6714/1171/7216/Functions_and_Minimum_Standards_forNational_Reference_Laboratories_in_the_SADC_Region.pdf

21. Shamsuzzaman AK. Role of National Reference Laboratory: Bangladesh perspective. Bangladesh Journal of Infectious Diseases. 2020;7(1):1.

22. LGC Group. National Reference Laboratories [Internet]. England: LGC Limited. 2022. Available from www.lgcgroup.com/what-we-do/national-laboratory-and-government-roles/national-laboratory-roles/national-reference-laboratories/

23. EU Science Hub. AQUILA - role and tasks of National Reference Laboratories [Internet]. EU: Directorate-General for Communication. 2022. Available from https://ec.europa.eu/jrc/en/aquila/national-reference-laboratories-role-and-tasks

24. World Health Organization. External quality assurance assessment scheme (EQAAS) [Internet]. Geneva: WHO; 2009. Available from www.who.int/teams/health-product-and-policy-standards/standards-and-specifications/norms-and-standards-for-pharmaceuticals/eqaas

25. World Health Organization. Overview of external quality assessment (EQA) [Internet]. Geneva: WHO. 2009. Available from www.who.int/publications/m/item/overview-of-external-quality-assessment-eqa

26. US Food and Drug Administration. What we do [Internet]. Silver Spring, MD: USFDA. 2022. Available from www.fda.gov/about-fda/what-we-do

27. Reddy GT, Reddy GN. Significance of pharmaceutical regulatory bodies-a review. PharmaTutor. 2017;5(8):15–22.

28. US Food and Drug Administration. Center for Biologics Evaluation and Research (CBER) [Internet]. Silver Spring, MD: USFDA; 2022. Available from www.fda.gov/about-fda/fda-organization/center-biologics-evaluation-and-research-cber

29. Central Drugs Laboratory. ABOUT [Internet]. Kasauli: CDSCO. 2022. Available from https://cdlkasauli.gov.in/CDL_KASAULI/Homepage

30. Wikipedia contributors. Central Drugs Standard Control Organisation (CDSCO) [Internet]. Wikipedia, 2023. Available from https://en.wikipedia.org/wiki/Central_Drugs_Standard_Control_Organisation

31. Central Drugs Standard Control Organization. About CDSCO [Internet]. Delhi CDSCO. 2022. Available from https://cdsco.gov.in/opencms/opencms/en/Home/

32. Suke SG, Kosta P, Negi H. Role of pharmacovigilance in India: an overview. Online Journal of Public Health Informatics. 2015;7(2):e223.

33. Kalaiselvan V, Thota P, Singh GN. Pharmacovigilance Programme of India: recent developments and future perspectives. Indian Journal of Pharmacology. 2016;48(6):624.

34. Indian Pharmacopoeia Commission (IPC). About IPC [Internet]. Ghaziabad: IPC. 2022. Available from http://ipc.gov.in/#skltbsResponsive1

35. Indian Pharmacopoeia Commission (IPC). Mission and vision of IPC [Internet]. Ghaziabad: IPC. 2022. Available from http://ipc.gov.in/about-us/about-ipc/mission-vision-and-objectives-of-ipc.html

36. Singh, & Associates. India: Indian Pharmacopoeia Commission (IPC) releases eighth edition of Indian Pharmacopoeia (IP) [Internet]. Mondaq AI: 2018. Available from www.mondaq.com/india/food-and-drugs-law/671182/indian-pharmacopoeia-commission-ipc-releases-eighth-edition-of-indian-pharmacopoeia-ip

37. National Health Portal (NHP). National Formulary of India [Internet]. MoHFW. 2015. Available from www.nhp.gov.in/national-formulary-of-india_mtl#:~:text=11035%2F2%2F06%2D%20DFQC,of%20Health%20and%20Family%20Welfare

38. GK Today. National Formulary of India [Internet]. 2015. Available from www.gktoday.in/topic/national-formulary-of-india/

39. Indian Pharmacopoeia Commission (IPC). National Formulary of India (NFI) [Internet]. Ghaziabad: IPC. 2022. Available from www.ipc.gov.in/#skltbsResponsive3

40. Indian Pharmacopoeia Commission (IPC). IP- Reference Substances (IPRS) [Internet]. Ghaziabad: IPC; 2022. Available from www.ipc.gov.in/#skltbsResponsive4

41. Indian Pharmacopoeia Commission (IPC). Analytical Research and Development ((AR&D) [Internet]. Ghaziabad: IPC. 2022. Available from www.ipc.gov.in/#skltbsResponsive5

42. Indian Pharmacopoeia Commission (IPC). Quality Assurance (QA) [Internet]. Ghaziabad: IPC. 2022. Available from www.ipc.gov.in/#skltbsResponsive7

43. Central Research Institute. About us [Internet]. Kasauli: Central Research Institute Kasauli; 2022. Available from https://crikasauli.nic.in/

44. National Institute of Biologicals. Welcome to NIB [Internet]. Noida:NIB. 2022. Available from www.nib.gov.in/homepage.aspx

45. National Institute of Biologicals. Quality Policy [Internet].Noida: NIB. 2022. Available from www.nib.gov.in/quality.aspx

4 Accreditations for Biologicals

Manjula Kiran
National Institute of Biologicals, Ministry of Health and
Family Welfare, Government of India, A-32, Sector-62,
Noida – 201309, India

4.1 BACKGROUND

The concepts of quality assurance (QA) and quality control (QC) have now been encompassed by the concept of a quality management system. QA addresses issues ranging from the sample collection in the laboratory to the reporting of test results, whereas QC comprises an assessment of whether the procedure is performed in accordance with specifications. The International Organization for Standardization (ISO) 15189 [1, 2] is the internationally recognized standard for quality management systems.

The main benefit achieved from adopting the laboratory quality management system (LQMS) is improved management in terms of better work and resource allocation, including foreseeing the possible circumstances and tasks. However, for laboratories with no accreditation experience, preparation, and presentation for ISO:17025 [3] may seem to be long and time-consuming [4].

Trust, competitiveness, better efficiency, teamwork, and quality improvement awareness are some of the other advantages achieved by accepting a standard, which results in better service and acceptance of testing and calibration results [5, 6]. Standards can also serve as a helping guide to the laboratory staff to achieve accreditation [7]. Accreditation is a critical way to address knowledge, budget, planning, policy, and staff required for improved laboratory services [8].

4.2 NATIONAL ACCREDITATION BOARD FOR TESTING AND CALIBRATION LABORATORIES (NABL)

The International Organization for Standardization (ISO) has developed an international standard, ISO/IEC 17025, "General requirements for the competence of testing and calibration laboratories" designed specifically for testing and calibration laboratories. It started as Guide ISO/IEC 25, which later was upgraded to standard ISO/IEC 17025. The standard was initially developed for industrial laboratories, such as biological, chemical, electrical, electronics, mechanical, photometry, and thermal but was later applied to clinical laboratories as well (ISO/

DOI: 10.1201/9781032697444-4

IEC 17025:2005). This led to interpretation problems, and hence a closely related standard, namely ISO 15189 "Medical Laboratories – Particular Requirements for Quality and Competence" was developed specifically for clinical laboratories using language in harmony with the medical testing environment with the objective of giving quality service to patients and healthcare providers (ISO 15189:2007). The ISO/IEC 17025 and ISO 15189 standards are being used around the globe by many accreditation bodies, including the International Laboratory Accreditation Cooperation (ILAC).

Accreditation can simply be defined as the formal recognition, authorization, and registration of a laboratory demonstrating the capability, competence, and credibility to carry out the tasks that it intends to do. It is also vital as it provides feedback to laboratories on whether the work they are performing is in accordance with the international criteria for technical competence. A third-party certification is provided to the laboratory through accreditation, saying that the laboratory is competent to perform the specific test or type of test. Laboratory accreditation is also a means to improve customer confidence to accept the test reports issued by the laboratory [9].

As defined clearly by International Organization for Standardization (ISO), accreditation is a third-party attestation related to a conformity assessment body conveying a formal demonstration of its competence to carry out specific conformity tasks (IEC 17000:2004). Accordingly, the laboratory's competence is assessed for the tests in its scope and the laboratory's compliance with the stated quality management system (QMS). It, thus, endorses the QMS of the audited laboratory.

As defined by the World Health Organization, accreditation is a comprehensive evaluation of the critical systems that make up a healthcare establishment and is an increasingly projected method for enhancing quality at the healthcare delivery level [10, 11]. Although the developed countries, especially in the western hemisphere, were early adopters of healthcare accreditation, during the last decade, accreditation for healthcare systems has also been aggressively promoted in developing countries, such as India [12].

In India, for clinical care and research laboratories, which have not opted for accreditation, the Indian Council of Medical Research (ICMR) has implemented easy-to-follow WHO-developed policies and procedures: Guidelines on Good Clinical Laboratory Practices (GCLP) [13] as a step toward quality improvement. In the African region, the Stepwise Laboratory Quality Improvement Process Towards Accreditation (SLIPTA) and the Strengthening Laboratory Management Toward Accreditation (SLMTA) have helped in achieving quality diagnostic services (the WHO guide for the Stepwise Laboratory Improvement Process Towards Accreditation (SLIPTA) in the African region. SLIPTA offers a checklist for improving the quality of public health laboratories to achieve the requirements of the ISO 15189 standard, enabling the laboratories to develop and document their ability to detect, identify, and promptly report all diseases of public health significance. SLMTA is a systematic quality improvement program on implementing practical quality management systems in resource-limited settings using available resources. It was created by the US Centers for Disease Control and Prevention in collaboration with the WHO Regional Office for Africa, the Clinton Health Access Initiative, and the American Society for Clinical Pathology [2].

4.2.1 IMPORTANCE OF NABL IN QUALITY CONTROL REGULATION

As per the document NABL 100 – "General Information Brochure" [14], published by NABL for guidance regarding NABL accreditation and its procedure, accreditation provides formal recognition of competent conformity assessment bodies (CABs), providing customers with reliable testing (including medical), calibration, proficiency testing, and reference material producer services. This in turn enhances customer confidence in accepting the testing/calibration reports issued by accredited laboratories. Furthermore, the competence of accredited laboratories at international levels is also essential for the globalization of the Indian economy and the liberalization policies initiated by the Government in reducing trade barriers and providing greater thrust to exports.

In brief, some of the benefits of accreditation (Figure 4.1) of a conformity assessment body by NABL in accordance with the international standard are as follows:

- Robust quality management system and continual improvement: Better control of laboratory operations and feedback to laboratories as to whether they have sound quality assurance systems and are technically competent.

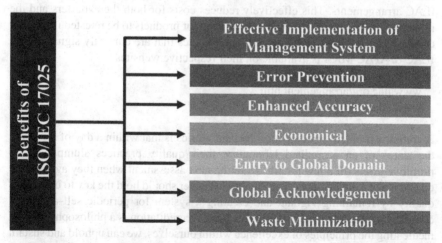

FIGURE 4.1 Benefits of adopting ISO IEC 17025. The various benefits of ISO/IEC 17025 include access to the global marketplace, international recognition, a sound management system, preventing defects, increased accuracy, cost savings, reduced waste, etc.

- Assurance for accurate and reliable results: the results from accredited laboratories are used extensively by regulators for the public benefit in providing services that promote an unpolluted environment, safe food, clean water, energy, health, and social care services.
- Better customer confidence and satisfaction in testing/calibration reports.
- Access to the global market and international recognition/equivalence: users of accredited laboratories enjoy greater access for their products in domestic and international markets. Accredited laboratories receive international recognition, allowing their data and results to be more readily accepted in overseas markets. Accreditation helps to reduce costs for manufacturers and exporters, who have their products or materials tested in accredited laboratories, by reducing or eliminating the need for retesting in another country.
- Helpful in participating in tenders that require independently verified laboratories.
- Savings in terms of time and money due to reducing or eliminating the need for retesting products.

NABL accreditation also helps the laboratories to reach global customers as NABL is a signatory to ILAC and APAC Mutual Recognition Arrangements (MRA). Such international arrangements facilitate acceptance of the test/calibration results between countries to which MRA partners represent. This developing system of international mutual recognition agreements between accreditation bodies has enabled accredited laboratories to achieve international recognition and allowed test data accompanying exported goods to be readily accepted on overseas markets amongst the countries which have already qualified as significant to ILAC arrangements. This effectively reduces costs for both the exporters and the importers, as it reduces or eliminates the need for products to be retested in another country. The information on accreditation bodies that are currently signatories to ILAC & APAC MRA is available on their respective websites:

www.ilac.org/arrangement.htm
www.apac.org/apac_mra.html

A common problem with most of the laboratories is that within a day of receiving the status of an accredited laboratory, their quality practices slump back to primitive levels till a few months from the next assessment when they again wake up and make a quality dash. The Quality Manager should hold the key to upholding quality by remaining vigilant and creating a system for periodic self-audit and continuous laboratory technology education. Accreditation is a philosophy, and by inculcating the principles of excellence within ourselves, we can uphold and sustain the quality and the accredited status of our laboratories [15]. Thankfully, NABL accreditation is not a one-time phenomenon. Once a laboratory gets accredited, accreditation is generally valid for 2 years. On application from the laboratory, for renewal of accreditation at least 6 months before the expiry of the validity period of accreditation, NABL conducts periodical surveillance of the CAB on annual basis.

4.2.2 DOCUMENTS REQUIRED FOR NABL ACCREDITATION

General requirements for the competence of testing and calibration laboratories, ISO/IEC 17025, Third edition, 2017-11, describes the following requirements as general requirements (clause 4), structural requirements (clause 5), resource requirements (clause 6), process requirements (clause 7), and management system requirements (clause 8), along with the scope, normative references, and terms & conditions. There are a total of 8 clauses and 28 subclauses, according to which the laboratory must prepare the documents to undergo accreditation process.

The clauses and subclauses are mentioned below in detail:

CLAUSE 4: GENERAL REQUIREMENTS

- **Clause 4.1 (Impartiality)** – Laboratory management shall be committed to impartiality and ensure that all the activities in the laboratory are undertaken impartially. Risks to impartiality shall be identified, and the laboratory shall be able to eliminate or minimize such risks.
- **Clause 4.2 (Confidentiality)** – Through legally enforceable commitments, the laboratory shall be responsible for all the information obtained during laboratory activities. The customer shall be informed, in advance, of any information made available by the laboratory in the public domain. Any other information shall be considered proprietary information and shall be regarded as confidential.

CLAUSE 5: STRUCTURAL REQUIREMENTS

- **Clause 5.1** – The laboratory shall be a legal entity or a defined part of a legal entity and is legally responsible for its activities.
- **Clause 5.2** – Management shall have overall responsibility for the laboratory.
- **Clause 5.3** – The laboratory activities shall be defined and documented, excluding the externally provided laboratory activities on an ongoing basis.
- **Clause 5.4** – Laboratory activities shall be carried out in such a way as to meet the requirements of this document, the laboratory's customers, regulatory authorities, and organizations providing recognition. This shall include laboratory activities performed in all its permanent facilities, sites away from its permanent facilities, associated temporary or mobile facilities, or at a customer's facility.
- **Clause 5.5** – Organizational and management structure of the laboratory shall be well defined along with the responsibility, authority, and interrelationship of all personnel who manage, perform, or verify the laboratory activities. The procedures shall be documented to the extent to ensure the consistent application of its activities and the validity of the results.

- **Clause 5.6** – The laboratory shall have personnel who have the authority and resources to carry out their duties, including implementation, maintenance, and improvement of the management system, to identify any deviations from the management system or from the procedures, to initiate actions to prevent or minimize such deviations, to report the management on the performance or any need for improvement and ensuring the effectiveness of laboratory activities.
- **Clause 5.7** – Laboratory management shall ensure that communication regarding the effectiveness and integrity of the management system occur when management system changes are planned and implemented.

CLAUSE 6: RESOURCE REQUIREMENTS

- **Clause 6.1 (General)** – The laboratory shall be well-equipped with personnel, facilities, equipment, systems, and support services necessary to manage and perform its laboratory activities.
- **Clause 6.2 (Personnel)** – All laboratory personnel shall act impartially, be competent, and work according to the laboratory's management system. They shall fulfill the requirements for education, qualification, training, technical knowledge, skills, and experience and shall document their competence requirements for each functioning of the laboratory. They shall also be able to evaluate the significance of deviations if any. Duties and responsibilities of the personnel shall be communicated through management. Thus, the procedures and records for the personnel competence requirements, selection, training, supervision, and authorization shall be retained in the laboratory. Development, modification, verification, and validation of methods, analysis of results, report, review, and authorization of results shall be carried out by authorized personnel only.
- **Clause 6.3 (Facilities and environmental conditions)** – The validity of results shall not be affected by the facilities and environmental conditions maintained by the laboratory. The necessary facilities and environmental requirements shall be documented. Environmental conditions in accordance with relevant specifications, methods, or procedures shall be monitored, controlled, and recorded along with the implementation and monitoring of measures to control facilities.
- **Clause 6.4 (Equipment)** – The laboratory shall be well-equipped with equipment (including measuring instruments, software, measurement standards, reference materials, reference data, reagents, consumables, or auxiliary apparatus) required for performing laboratory activities. Procedures for handling, transport, storage, use, and maintenance of equipment shall be in place in order to ensure their proper functioning. Before being placed into service, the equipment shall conform to the specified requirements per the laboratory activities. Measurement accuracy and/or measurement uncertainty of the equipment used for measurement shall be considered to provide a

valid result. A periodic calibration program of the measuring equipment shall be in place to establish the metrological traceability of the results. Periodic calibration of equipment shall be taken up to establish metrological traceability and/or when the measurement accuracy or uncertainty affects the validity of the reported results. The laboratory shall review the calibration program to maintain confidence in the status of calibration. All equipment calibrated/requiring calibration shall be labeled or coded to allow the user to clearly identify the calibration status of the equipment. Out-of-order equipment affecting the test results shall be clearly labeled and taken out of service until it has been verified to perform correctly. Intermediate checks shall be performed, wherever necessary, to maintain confidence in the performance of the equipment. Reference values and correction factors shall be updated and implemented wherever required. The laboratory shall prevent unintended adjustments of equipment. Records about identity, manufacturer details, serial number, location, IQ/OQ/PQ records, calibration details, maintenance plan, damages/malfunction/modification/repair (if any) of the equipment shall be maintained by the laboratory.

- **Clause 6.5 (Metrological traceability)** – Metrological traceability of the quantitative results shall be maintained, taking into consideration the calibrations that may contribute to MU (measurement uncertainty). Measurement results shall be traceable to the International System of Units (SI), wherever possible, either through calibration provided by a competent laboratory or the use of certified reference materials provided by a competent producer with stated metrological traceability to the SI or directly comparing with national or international standards. Where the traceability to the SI units is not technically possible, the laboratory shall demonstrate metrological traceability to an appropriate reference.

- **Clause 6.6 (Externally provided products and services)** – The laboratory shall use only suitable externally provided products and services. Procedures and records related to review and approval of the laboratory's requirements for externally provided products and services, criteria for evaluation, selection, monitoring of performance and reevaluation of the external providers, conformance of externally provided products and services the laboratory's requirements, etc., shall be retained by the laboratory. In addition, clear communication shall be made to external service and product providers regarding the products and services to be provided, acceptance criteria, competence, and activities that the laboratory, or its customer, intends to perform at the external provider's premises.

CLAUSE 7: PROCESS REQUIREMENTS

- **Clause 7.1 (Review of requests, tenders and contracts)** – The procedure for the review of requests, tenders, and contracts shall be written in a way to ensure that the requirements are adequately defined, documented, and understood and also the appropriate methods or procedures are selected and are capable of meeting the customers' needs. The decision rule shall be communicated to the customer. Also, a statement of conformity to specification or standard for the test or calibration shall be provided to the customer, when requested.

- **Clause 7.2 (Selection, verification and validation of methods)** –
  - Selection and verification of methods: Appropriate methods and procedures for all laboratory activities shall be used, and, where appropriate, measurement uncertainty, and statistical techniques for analysis of data shall be used. Updated/latest valid version of methods, procedures, and supporting documentation, such as instructions, standards, manuals, and reference data relevant to the laboratory activities, shall be used and readily available to personnel. Unless specified by the customer, the methods published either in international, regional, or national standards, by reputable technical organizations, or in relevant scientific texts or journals, or as specified by the equipment manufacturer, are recommended. Laboratory-developed or modified methods can also be used. The development of a new method shall be taken as a planned activity by the competent personnel. Validation records of methods shall be retained before introducing the method to perform laboratory activities. On the revision of the method by the issuing body, verification needs to be performed again. Any deviation from the method shall be documented and authorized.
  - Validation of methods: Non-standard/laboratory-developed methods shall be validated. A new method validation shall be taken up in the case of changes made to a validated method. The laboratory shall retain records for validation procedure, specifications, performance characteristics, and results.
- **Clause 7.3 (Sampling)** – A sampling plan and method shall be in place to carry out the sampling of substances, materials, or products for subsequent testing or calibration. The sampling method shall describe the selection of samples, sampling plan, sample preparation, etc., and all such records related to sampling shall be retained by the laboratory.
- **Clause 7.4 (Handling of test or calibration items)** – Procedure for the transportation, receipt, handling, protection, storage, retention, and disposal or return of test or calibration items including the precautions to be taken to avoid deterioration, contamination, loss or damage to the item during handling, transporting, storing/waiting, and preparation for testing or calibration shall be well documented. Any deviation noticed at the time of receipt of the test or calibration item shall be recorded, and the laboratory shall inform the customer about further instructions before proceeding. Specific environmental conditions required for storage shall be maintained and monitored.
- **Clause 7.5 (Technical records)** – Technical records for each laboratory activity shall contain the results, report, and sufficient information to

facilitate, measurement uncertainty (if applicable). It should also bear details regarding the date, name of the performer, original observations, data, and calculations. Amendments shall be traceable to the previous or original version, including dates and authorizations for the alterations.

- **Clause 7.6 (Evaluation of measurement uncertainty, MU)** – Measurement uncertainty shall be identified by the laboratory while testing and calibration. MU shall be calculated for all calibrations of the equipment.

- **Clause 7.7 (Ensuring the validity of results)** – The laboratory shall have a procedure for monitoring the validity of results. The trends in the resulting data shall be detectable. This monitoring shall be planned and reviewed and shall include details, such as reference materials, working standards, alternative instrumentation, intermediate equipment checks, retest/replicate testing using the same or different methods, intralaboratory comparisons, testing of blind samples, etc. Where available, the performance of the laboratory shall also be monitored by comparison with results of other laboratories by participation in the proficiency testing initiated by the proficiency testing providers competent as per the requirements mentioned in ISO/IEC 17043. Data from such monitoring activities shall be analyzed and used to improve laboratory activities.

- **Clause 7.8 (Reporting of results)** – All the results shall be reviewed and authorized before release such that accurate, clear, unambiguous, and objective results are presented in a report in a simplified way.

As per NABL accreditation requirements, the general and common details to be mentioned in the report shall include title, name, and address of the laboratory, location of performance (e.g., name of the department), unique identification number (e.g., file no. or analytical report number) customer information, date of receipt of test/calibration item, the method used, date of performance, date of issue of the report, results with the unit of measurement (if applicable), authorizations and a statement to the effect that relate only to the items tested, calibrated, or sampled and that the report shall not be reproduced without approval, etc. Also, where the laboratory is not involved in sampling (e.g., the sample has been provided by the customer), the report shall clearly state that the results apply to the sample as received. However, if the laboratory is responsible for sampling, the report shall include the date of sampling, unique ID issued to the item, location of sampling, reference to sampling method, etc. Specific requirements for test reports shall include information on test conditions, statement of conformity or specifications, measurement uncertainty (if applicable), opinions, and interpretations.

For laboratories involved in calibration services, the calibration certificates shall include the MU of the measurement result, the conditions (e.g., environmental) under which the calibrations were made, metrological traceability, a statement of conformity or specifications, opinions, and interpretations. While reporting the results, the decision rule shall be implied along with a statement of conformity to a specification or standard. Only authorized personnel shall express the statements about opinions and interpretations, and these should be based on the results obtained from the tested or the calibrated item. The laboratory shall maintain records of any such opinions and interpretations. While issuing any amendments to the issued reports, the change shall be clearly identified, including the reason for the change. If issued after amendment, the new report shall be uniquely identified and contain a reference to the original that it replaces.

- **Clause 7.9 (Complaints)** – The process to receive, evaluate, and make decisions on complaints shall be documented by the laboratory such that it contains details regarding the description of the complaint, tracking, and action taken on the complaint. In addition, a formal notice shall be handed to the complainant regarding the end of the complaint.
- **Clause 7.10 (Nonconforming work)** – The procedure shall be implemented in the laboratory if any laboratory activity does not conform to its procedures and requirements. The procedure shall clearly define the responsibility, authority, actions taken to impact results, etc. All such records of non-conforming work and actions shall be retained in the laboratory. Corrective action shall be implemented where the evaluation indicates that the non-conforming work could recur.
- **Clause 7.11 (Control of data and information management)** – The laboratory shall have access to the data and information needed to perform laboratory activities. Collection, processing, recording, reporting, storage, or retrieval of data shall be validated using laboratory information management system(s). In the case of changes in laboratory software, etc., the same shall be authorized, validated, and documented before implementation.

    Only authorized personnel shall be able to access the laboratory information management system(s), and be safeguarded against tempering, including recording failures and corrective actions taken. In addition, instructions, manuals, and reference data relevant to the laboratory information management system(s) shall be readily available to personnel.

CLAUSE 8: MANAGEMENT SYSTEM REQUIREMENTS

- **Clause 8.1 (Options)** – Management systems capable of supporting and assuring the quality of laboratory results shall be established and maintained in accordance with Option A or B mentioned in the NABL document. Option A states that the laboratory's management system shall address documentation, control of the document, records, improvement, corrective action, internal audits, management reviews, etc., as mentioned in subclauses 8.2–8.9. Option B states that in addition to the requirements mentioned in Option A, the management system shall also be in accordance with the provisions of ISO 9001.
- **Clause 8.2 (Management system documentation)** – Policies and objectives addressing competence and impartiality are acknowledged and implemented

at all levels of the laboratory organization by the laboratory management system.

Laboratory management shall take care of commitment to development, implementation, and continual improvement. All personnel involved in laboratory activities shall have access to the parts of the management system documentation and related information that are applicable to their responsibilities.

- **Clause 8.3 (Control of management system documents)** – All approved documents (internal and external) shall be controlled, periodically reviewed, and updated. Documents should be uniquely identified with the current version available at the point of use. The use of obsolete documents should be prevented.

- **Clause 8.4 (Control of records)** – Controls needed for the identification, storage, protection, back-up, archive, retrieval, retention time, and disposal of its records shall be implemented by the laboratory, and access to these records shall fulfill the confidentiality commitments; however, the records shall be readily available to the authorized personnel.

- **Clause 8.5 (Actions to address risks and opportunities)** – Actions shall be taken to address risks and opportunities to provide assurance to the management system, reduce the risk of potential failures, and achieve improvement.

- **Clause 8.6 (Improvement)** – The laboratory shall identify opportunities for improvement and their implementation. Customer feedback, positive or negative, shall be sought and analyzed by the laboratory to improve the management system, laboratory activities, and customer service.

- **Clause 8.7 (Corrective actions)** – In case of non-conformity, the laboratory shall take action and address the consequences. The laboratory shall determine the causes of the non-conformity by reviewing and analyzing it to ensure the elimination of the reason for the non-conformity. To ensure that the non-conformity is not repeated, the laboratory shall take effective corrective action.

- **Clause 8.8 (Internal audits)** – The laboratory shall conduct internal audits at planned intervals to ensure that the management system is effectively implemented and maintained. The frequency, methods, responsibilities, planning requirements, and reporting shall be maintained as the audit program defining the audit scope, results of the audit, corrective actions, etc.

- **Clause 8.9 (Management reviews)** – Similar to the internal audits, the laboratory management shall be reviewed at planned intervals to ensure its continuing suitability, adequacy, and effectiveness. Records related to the policies, outcome of the recent audits, assessment of external bodies, customer feedback, complaints, risk identification, other relevant factors such as training, etc. The management review shall record all decisions and actions related to its effectiveness, improvement, or any change required.

4.3   THE CENTRAL DRUGS LABORATORY

Drugs & Cosmetic Act & Rules 1940 (16) & 1945 define the following functions
for the Central Drugs Laboratory:
   It states that the laboratory shall

   (i)   analyze or test such samples of drugs as may be sent to it under subsection
         (2) of section 11 or under subsection (4) of section 25 of the Act;
   (ii) carry out such other duties as may be entrusted to it by the Central
         Government or, with the permission of the Central Government, by a State
         Government after consultation with the Drugs Technical Advisory Board.

Likewise, the Central Research Institute, Kasauli, shall function in respect of the
following drugs or classes of drugs:

   (1) Sera
   (2) Solution of serum proteins intended for injection
   (3) Vaccines
   (4) Toxins
   (5) Antigens
   (6) Antitoxins
   (7) Sterilized surgical ligature and sterilized surgical suture
   (8) Bacteriophages

Functions pertaining to the testing of Oral Polio Vaccine shall be exercised by the
Deputy Director and Head of the Polio Vaccine Testing Laboratory in the case of
the Central Research Institute, Kasauli, and Directors of Pasteur Institute of India,
Coonoor, Enterovirus Research Centre (Indian Council of Medical Research),
Mumbai and National Institute of Biologicals, Noida.
   Indian Veterinary Research Institute, Izatnagar shall exercise the functions
of (1) antisera for veterinary use, (2) vaccines for veterinary use, (3) toxoids for
veterinary use, and (4) diagnostic antigens for veterinary use.
   Central Drugs Testing Laboratory, Chennai, shall exercise its function in respect
of the testing of condoms.
   Testing of VDRL antigen shall be exercised as function by the Laboratory of the
Serologist and Chemical Examiner to the Government of India, Calcutta, and shall
be performed by the Serologist and Chemical Examiner of the said laboratory.
   Testing of intrauterine sevices and Falope rings shall be carried out at the Central
Drugs Testing Laboratory, Thane, Maharashtra.
   The functions of the laboratory with respect to human blood and human blood
products, including components, to test for freedom of HIV antibodies shall be
carried out by the following institutes/hospitals:

   (a) National   Institute   for   Communicable   Disease,   Department   of
         Microbiology, Delhi.

(b) National Institute of Virology, Pune
(c) Centre of Advanced Research in Virology, Christian Medical College, Vellore.

Homoeopathy Pharmacopoeia Laboratory, Ghaziabad, shall function with respect to the testing of the homoeopathic medicines.

The functions in respect of the following kits or class of drugs shall be carried out at the National Institute of Biologicals, Noida:

(1) **Blood grouping reagents**
(2) **Diagnostic kits for human immunodeficiency virus, hepatitis B surface antigen, and hepatitis C virus**
(3) **Blood products**
    (a) Human albumin
    (b) Human normal immunoglobulin (intramuscular and intravenous)
    (c) Human coagulation factor VIII
    (d) Human coagulation factor IX
    (e) Plasma protein fractionation
    (f) Fibrin sealant kit
    (g) Anti inhibitor coagulation complex
(4) **Recombinant products**
    (a) Recombinant insulin and insulin analogue
    (b) r-erythropoietin (EPO)
    (c) r-granulocyte colony-stimulating factor (G-CSF)
(5) **Biochemical kits**
    (a) Glucose test strips
    (b) Fully automated analyzer-based glucose reagents

REFERENCES

1. ISO 15189:2007. International Organization for Standardization: ISO 15189 medical laboratories-particular requirements for quality and competence, 2007.
2. Pai S & Frater JL. Quality management and accreditation in laboratory hematology: perspectives from India. International Journal of Laboratory Hematology 2019;41(Suppl. 1):177–83.
3. ISO/IEC 17025: 2005. International Organization for Standardization: ISO/IEC 17025 general requirements for the competence of testing and calibration laboratories, 2005.
4. Macchi Silva VV & Ribeiro JLD. Obtaining laboratory accreditation-required activities. International Journal of Healthcare Quality Assurance 2019; 32(1): 71–83.
5. Vlachos NA, Michail C & Sotiropoulou D. Is ISO/IEC 17025 accreditation a benefit or hindrance to testing laboratories? The Greek Experience; Journal of Food Composition and Analysis 2002;15(6):749–57.
6. Rodima A et al. ISO 17025 quality system in a university environment. Accreditation and Quality Assurance 2005;10(7):369–72.

7. Malkoc E & Neuteboom W. The current status of forensic science laboratory accreditation in Europe. Forensic Science International 2007;167(2–3):121–26.

8. Kanitvittaya S et al. Laboratory quality improvement in Thailand's northernmost provinces. International Journal of Health Care Quality Assurance 2010;23(1):22–34.

9. Kanagasabapathy A S & Rao P. Laboratory Accreditation-Procedural Guidelines. Indian Journal of Clinical Biochemistry 2005;20(2):186–8.

10. Al-Assaf AF, Sheikh M. Quality Improvement in Primary Healthcare: A Practical Guide. Geneva, Switzerland: World Health Organization: 2004.

11. World Health Organization. Quality and Accreditation in Health Care Services: A Global Review. Geneva, Switzerland: World Health Organization; 2003. Available from http://whqlibdoc.who.int/hq/2003/WHO_EIP_OSD_2003.1.pdf

12. Ajay K, Avinash P, Narayan M. Impact of accreditation on documentation and staff perception in the ophthalmology department of an Indian medical college. Indian Journal of Ophthamology 2021;69:337–42.

13. World Health Organization. Good Clinical Laboratory Practice (GCLP) Geneva, Switzerland: World Health Organization; 2009.

14. NABL 100- General requirements for the competence of testing and calibration laboratories INTERNATIONAL STANDARD, ISO/IEC 17025: 2017, Third edition.

15. Wadhwa V, Rai S, Thukral T, Chopra M. Laboratory quality management system: road to accreditation and beyond. Indian Journal of Medical Microbiology 2012;30(2):131–40.

16. The Drugs and Cosmetics Act and Rules: The Drugs and Cosmetics Act, 1940 (23 of 1940) (as amended up to the 31 December, 2016) and The Drugs and Cosmetics Rules, 1945 (as amended up to the 31 December, 2016).

5 Indian Industries and Biologicals

Archana Upadhyay, Ashrat Manzoor,
Brij Bhushan, and Shalini Tewari
National Institute of Biologicals, Sector-62, A-32,
Industrial Area, Noida, Uttar Pradesh – 201309, India

5.1 BACKGROUND

The three essential components supporting the contemporary healthcare sector are biologicals, e.g., vaccines, therapeutic antibodies, blood products, enzymes, hormones, and medical devices including in vitro diagnostic kits. Like vaccines and chemical-based drugs, medical devices are crucial for patient screening, monitoring, diagnosing, treating and facilitating patients restoring to their normal life. Biologicals are produced using a variety of biotechnological techniques, including recombinant deoxyribonucleic acid technology, regulated gene expression, and antibody technology from natural resources like animals, or microorganisms [1, 2]. Biologicals have established themselves as ground-breaking advancements in the pharmaceutical sector. By stopping the progression of the disease, reducing the symptoms, and enhancing the quality of life, biologicals have benefited patients with rheumatologic diseases, inflammatory bowel disease, malignant conditions, dermatological ailments, and other connective tissue disorders [3, 4]. One of the most popular drugs on the market today is biologic; however, due to its extremely high price, many patients find it unaffordable and inaccessible. This is especially true in developing nations, where a sizable portion of the population lives in poverty and the idea of health insurance is still in its infancy [5, 6].

The inventing company loses its intellectual property rights and patent protection after a predetermined period, but there is still a silver lining that creates a window of opportunity for different firms, companies and start-ups that can express interest in producing similar products at a lower cost [7]. The term "biosimilar" refers to a biologic product that is very similar to another biological product that has been approved by the Food and Drug Administration (FDA), also known as the "reference product," and that differs from the reference product in neither safety nor efficacy in any clinically significant ways [8]. However, due to the complicated structure of similar biologics, which may be influenced by minute changes in sequences and post-translational modifications, they are not completely identical to reference biologics. [9]. Medical professionals and experts are hopeful that the usage of biosimilars may lower the price of biologics and eventually improve patients' access to these life-saving medications [10]. The manufacture and marketing of biosimilars are carried out by more than 100 biopharmaceutical companies in India. Biosimilars are referred to as "similar biologics" by Indian regulatory agencies. Even though India was among the first nations in the world to adopt it, there was no clear guideline for "similar biologics," and the approval process for these products is more onerous and demands more information than that for other generic medications. The Central Drugs Standard Control Organization (CDSCO) to solve the problems and difficulties related to the development of similar biologics, created Guidelines on Similar Biologics; Regulatory Requirements for Marketing Authorization in India in partnership with the Department of Biotechnology (DBT) in 2012, and they were updated in 2016 [11–13]. These regulations cover the quality, safety, and effectiveness of comparable biologics as well as the control of the manufacturing process. It addresses the regulatory requirements for comparable biologics both before and after launch. The development of biologics and their preclinical testing are supervised by DBT through the Review Committee on Genetic Manipulation. Similar biologics are subjected to regulation in India as per the Drug and Cosmetic Act (1940), Drug and Cosmetic Rules, 1945, and Rules for Manufacture, Use, Import, Export, and Storage of Hazardous Microorganisms, Genetically Engineered Organisms or Cells, notified under Environmental (Protection) Act, 1986 [11].

In contrast to the previous requirement, which was that the reference biologic for which the biosimilar was to be developed had to be approved and marketed in India, CDSCO has made some significant revisions to its previous guideline. For example, the requirement is now either India or any other countries that are members of the International Council for Harmonization (i.e., Canada, European Union, Japan, Switzerland, and the United States). It also makes an effort to coordinate with other international organizations like the World Health Organization and European Medicine Agency (EMA). Indian guidelines state that biologics should be developed in a stepwise manner to demonstrate how closely a biosimilar product resembles reference products in terms of both molecular characteristics and quality. The emphasis on post-marketing studies, which CDSCO claims are meant "to further reduce the residual risk of the similar biologic," is another difference between the 2012 guidance and the document released in 2016. CDSCO has made it mandatory for the biopharmaceutical company to conduct a phase IV study with a minimum of 200 patients within 2 years of receiving of marketing approval [11]. To assure quality, safety, and efficacy as well as consistency with previous batches, each batch of a biotherapeutic product undergoes meticulous testing at each step of production. The adoption of WHO international reference standards facilitates further assuring the consistency of a product throughout the course of several batches and makes it possible to compare biologicals produced by different manufacturers and/or in different countries. The development of generic specifications, which govern raw materials, production, and regulatory control for many different product categories is a critical phase in this process.

5.1.1 BIOLOGICAL PRODUCTS

Biological products are regulated by the Food and Drug Administration (FDA) and are used to diagnose, prevent, treat, and cure diseases and medical conditions. Biological products are a diverse category of products and are generally large, complex molecules. These products may be produced through biotechnology in a living system, such as a microorganism, plant cell, or animal cell, and are often more difficult to characterize than small molecule drugs. The FDA regulates biological products that are used for diagnosis, prophylaxis, treatment, and eventually curing diseases and medical conditions. In general, biological products are large, complex molecules, and may be produced by biotechnology in a living system, such as a bacterium, plant cell, or animal cell. Therapeutic proteins (like filgrastim), monoclonal antibodies (like adalimumab), and vaccines (like those for influenza and tetanus) are just a few of the numerous biological products that have received approval in the United States. Characterizing and producing biological products can be difficult due to their nature, which can also include intrinsic variances brought on by the manufacturing process. These issues frequently do not arise in the creation of small-molecule medications. It is typical and anticipated throughout the manufacturing process for there to be small acceptable product variances across manufactured batches of the same biological product. The production procedure and the manufacturer's approach to managing product variances are both evaluated by the FDA as part of the evaluation process. These control measures are put in place to make sure that the product with consistent clinical performance is produced, by the manufacturers of biological products.

5.1.2 CONVENTIONAL DRUGS VS. BIOLOGICAL

Biologicals are a broad category that includes vaccines, blood and blood components, recombinant therapeutic proteins, allergens, somatic cells, and a broad spectrum of products that are isolated from natural sources viz. human, animal, or microbes. The process of manufacture is where biologicals and conventional pharmaceuticals diverge most. While biologics/biologicals are produced using biotechnological processes as opposed to conventional chemical synthesis, they require aseptic manufacturing practices from the very beginning of the manufacturing process (Figure 5.1). As a result, both time and money are heavily invested. For most conventional drugs, that is not the case. When compared to traditional medications, the majority of biologics are complicated mixes in terms of structure. The most effective treatment for a range of illnesses that were previously incurable with traditional chemical medications may one day be biologics, which are at the forefront of biomedical research. The complexity of evaluating the quality of biologicals compared to chemical drugs poses a challenge to the regulators (Table 5.1).

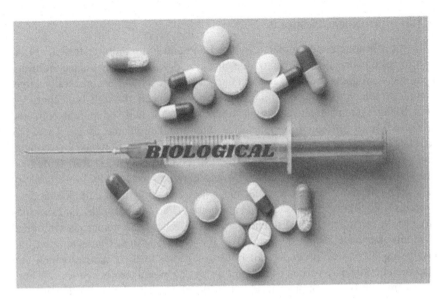

FIGURE 5.1   Conventional drugs and biologics.

TABLE 5.1
Major National Regulatory Agencies Worldwide

Country	Name of Regulatory Authority
India	Central Drug Standard Control Organization (CDSCO)
USA	Food and Drug Administration (FDA)
Europe	European Medicines Agency (EMA)
UK	Medicines and Healthcare Products Regulatory Agency (MHRA)
Australia	Therapeutic Goods Administration (TGA)
Canada	Health Canada
New Zealand	Medicines and Medical Devices Safety Authority (Medsafe)
China	State Food and Drug Administration (SFDA)
Japan	Ministry of Health, Labour & Welfare (MHLW)
Switzerland	SWISSMEDIC, Swiss Agency for Therapeutic Products

5.1.3   REFERENCE PRODUCT

The sole biological product, which has already received approval from a regulatory body, against which a proposed biosimilar or biological product is compared is known as a reference product [15]. A complete set of safety and efficacy data is among the criteria used to approve a reference product. To make sure a proposed biosimilar or biological product is substantially comparable to and devoid of clinically significant deviations from the reference product, the products are compared and assessed against one another.

5.1.4 BIOLOGICALS: GLOBAL SCENARIO

Regarding the worldwide market, the US FDA has already updated its regulations to remove the outmoded biologics requirement, allowing producers and inventors to investigate new technologies to increase the production of biologics [15]. The US FDA's ongoing regulatory updates for biologics clearance are anticipated to increase regulatory flexibility in the global pharmaceutical sector. Furthermore, the blockbuster biologics patents expiring and the government's efforts to lower healthcare costs by introducing biosimilars to the market are promoting excellence in the pharma and biotech sectors' ability to go global.

5.1.5 INDIAN BIOLOGICAL INDUSTRY

India has emerged as a global leader in the development of pharmaceuticals and biotechnology over the past few decades to the point where the nation is now referred to as the "Pharmacy" of the world. In 2019, the Indian biotechnology market was valued at US$ 63 billion and is anticipated to grow to US$ 150 billion by 2025 [16]. The global market for biologics is anticipated to escalate at a CAGR of 6% from US$ 253.41 billion in 2020 to US$ 268.51 billion in 2021. By 2025, the market can account for US$ 420.55 billion, growing at a CAGR of 12% [17]. Based on these figures, it is possible for the Indian biopharmaceutical sector and the bioservices to emerge as a major hub for biologics production, clinical trials, and contract research. The Indian pharmaceuticals market is distinctive in a number of ways: branded generics account for more than 70% of the retail market, and indigenous businesses have benefited from a dominating position thanks to early investments and formulation development skills. In terms of value, the Indian pharmaceuticals market is rated tenth globally, but it is ranked third in terms of the quantity of pharmaceutical items. According to a 2009 estimate by McKinsey, the Indian pharmaceutical business was worth $12.6 billion and is projected to grow to $100 billion by 2025, according to the Indian Brand Equity Foundation [16]. Leading Indian businesses are working hard to produce biologics and vaccines, including Biocon, Zydus Cadila, Bharat Biotech, and even the Serum Institute of India (SII). In 2006, patients in India received the first innovative biological treatment, a monoclonal antibody called BIOMab EGFR for head and neck cancer. The first biosimilar Herceptin to be created by Biocon and Mylan was CANMab, which was introduced in India in 2014. Thereafter, more biosimilar versions were created. The first Indian biosimilar to be commercialized in Japan was Insulin Glargine from Biocon in 2016. In December 2017, Ogivri, a biosimilar Trastuzumab co-developed by Biocon and Mylan, became the first biosimilar Herceptin to receive US approval. In 2018, Biocon and Mylan's co-developed biosimilar Fulphila (Pegfilgrastim) became the first biosimilar Neulasta to achieve

US approval. Fulphila subsequently turned into the first biosimilar created in India to be released for sale in the US in 2019. Indian pharmaceutical firms are in a good position to capitalize on the biosimilar industry and capture a sizeable portion of it over the coming 10 years. If handled correctly, this may be the Indian pharmaceutical industry's next success tale, following the tale of the generics in the US. The rising number of biosimilars already released by Indian businesses serves as a reminder of this potential. Opportunities provided by labor availability, industrial capabilities, and inexpensive development costs can significantly impact the Indian biologics industry in the years to come.

5.1.6 GOVERNMENT POLICIES FOR STRENGTHENING INDIAN BIOLOGICAL INDUSTRIES

India is looking into opportunities in biologicals and biosimilars to expand beyond generics because it is the "Global Generic Hub." Currently, simple biologicals like insulin, erythropoietin, medications for autoimmune and cardiovascular disease, and monoclonal antibodies are dominating the Indian biologicals market. The Indian medical device industry is on a fast development trajectory and has evolved tremendously over the past decade owing to the recent surge in demand, advances in regulation, and government support. With a variety of funding and investment strategies, the Indian government is encouraging the development of biotech-based drugs. The "Make in India" campaign initiatives are sufficient to benefit the Indian pharmaceutical industry. Some of the major governing bodies actively supporting India's biotech sector with various initiatives include the Department of Biotechnology (DBT), the Biotechnology Industry Research Assistance Council (BIRAC), the Union Health Ministry, and the Indian Council of Medical Research (ICMR). These organizations encourage Public Private Partnerships (PPP) to draw funding to the biotech industry. India is among the first nations to establish a department specifically for the biotechnology sector. In addition, the Department has established BIRAC, a non-profit organization, to support and enable developing biotechnology businesses to engage in strategic research and innovation by guiding them from conception to the commercialization of their products/technologies.

For years, policymakers have been debating how to give an impetus to manufacturing in India and make India a Global Manufacturing Hub. The "Make in India" program was recently introduced in order to promote investment, encourage innovation, improve talent development, safeguard intellectual property, and create world-class manufacturing infrastructure. The "Make in India" project is built upon four pillars that have been identified as having the potential to stimulate entrepreneurship in India across a variety of industries, not only the manufacturing one. According to "Make in India," "ease of doing business" is the single most crucial aspect in fostering entrepreneurship. Numerous actions have already been done to improve the business climate. The goal is to delicense and deregulate the sector throughout a company's entire lifecycle. A crucial condition for the development of the industry is the availability of modern, helpful infrastructure. In order to provide infrastructure based on cutting-edge technology with contemporary high-speed communication and integrated logistical arrangements, the government plans to construct industrial corridors and smart cities. By upgrading the infrastructure in industrial clusters, the current infrastructure will be enhanced. Fast-paced registration systems assist innovation and research activities, hence the infrastructure for intellectual property rights' registration setup has been updated. It is necessary to determine the skills that are needed by the industry and to develop the workforce accordingly.

Under the Make India initiative, a number of initiatives aimed at making doing business in India simpler have also been introduced. New IT-driven applications and tracking processes are taking the place of paperwork and bureaucracy. Several new initiatives have been initiated to rationalize and streamline licensing laws at the state government level, bringing them into compliance with international best practices.

The biotechnology sector has shown very positive growth during the past few years. This was largely because of a solid basis that was built over several decades, ranging from research and education to translation and product development. A concerted effort has been undertaken to interact with all stakeholders and introduce important policy changes that will serve as significant facilitators and drivers for this ecosystem, in addition to offering financial support. Over the past 20 years, efforts have been made to establish a strong enabling environment to support the expansion of the industry and to guarantee that the innovations and products generated through the intervention of cutting-edge frontier biotechnologies are provided in the service of human kind. The nation is undergoing significant adjustments to support the expansion of this industry. About 60% of the industry is focused on applications in human health, 10% on applications in agricultural biotechnology, and 30% on applications in industry, bioinformatics, and genomics.

5.1.7 THE REGULATORY PERSPECTIVE

The creation of biological products needs a sizable time and financial commitment. The regulatory procedure for biologicals approval in India is lengthy and requires numerous clearance phases, which might make it difficult for new breakthroughs in the sector to reach the market. The following are some ideas that can be used to maximize opportunities for Indian biologicals in the market [18].

i.   Establishing a powerful regulatory agency will allow for the achievement of the need for autonomy in policymaking and implementation.
ii. To speed up these legal procedures, a fast-track cell is needed to prevent market entrance delays caused by unclear subject matter, agreements, or SOPs.
iii. Increasing the capabilities and expertise of regulatory body reviewers can significantly impact the steps taken to approve biologics in India. In order to speed up the regulatory processes, periodic policy reviews are also obligatory.

Following the clearance of the first similar biologic in early 2000, the usage of biosimilars or similar biologics has grown in recent years. Despite the local regulatory environment, Indian firms like Biocon have achieved success on the global stage in partnership with Mylan by producing two biosimilar drugs: trastuzumab and pegfilgrastim. Due to the high expenses of litigation and regulations, the majority of Indian companies that manufacture biosimilars and biologicals choose not to access the international market.

5.2 STATUTORY REQUIREMENTS FOR QUALITY CONTROL REGULATION OF THERAPEUTICS

A key tool for drug regulation is manufacturer-independent quality control testing. The necessity for analysis should always be carefully taken into account because it does, however, necessitate a significant amount of resources. When considered from the standpoint of public health, independent quality control testing ought to be done if it adds value to the evaluation done and does not unnecessarily slow down patient access to medications. Safeguarding public health through the management of risk to quality should be given top priority. The medicines that are more likely to pose risks to patients should be the focus of testing, like those

- whose production is by manufacturers for whom there is insufficient proof of compliance with Good Manufacturing Practice (GMP) guidelines or whose provenance is unclear
- with suspicion of falsification
- which are assumed to be substandard due to improper distribution, storage practices, or instability
- which are suspicious of generating adverse reactions as a result of a quality issue
- whose analytical test results are required as proof in court

Regulators may conduct independent post-production testing for a variety of reasons and at different regulatory stages of the drug's lifecycle. When thinking about testing strategies, keep the following in mind.

- Preregistration testing of samples submitted for registration – the sample may not accurately reflect the quality of the product because it was chosen by the manufacturer. In some rare instances where data reviewers have some reservations, testing at this step may be helpful to determine the effectiveness of analytical procedures under local conditions.
- Official batch release of some biological products by the National Medicines Regulatory Authority (NMRA) – typically, this is required to comply with national regulations for particular products and are mentioned in guidelines.
- Premarketing evaluation of all or particular batches – it is common practice to collect samples of imported medicines at entrance points of a country. It would be appropriate to screen them and choose only those for testing that

exhibit physical indicators of instability or degradation, other signs of poor quality, or those whose origin is doubtful. In principle, the registration process should assure the quality of medicines, thus routine testing of every imported batch is not thought to be practical. Batch-to-batch testing may be valuable in certain circumstances, like in cases when it is not possible to perform a proper assessment for registration and verify conformity with good practices in production and/or product development. Prior to selecting whether to test a given product, the risk of substandard quality should be evaluated.

- Post-marketing testing as the initiative for risk-based sampling and surveillance/monitoring – the benefit of this strategy is choosing samples that are in the supply chain and are meant for patient administration.

The Indian NRA, CDSCO, is dynamic and robust to handle the issues posed by the country's sporadic introduction or development of newer biologicals. A highly specialized laboratory infrastructure (NCL) supported by an in vivo testing facility (animal house) with knowledge and experience gained from independent quality control testing is vital for undertaking the testing of biologicals because of their complexity, difficulty in characterization, and inherent variability from batch to batch. Additionally, NCL testing upholds a level of independent knowledge and expertise in test methodology, which is a crucial component of an NCL's general competency in terms of its capacity to efficiently monitor the product. CDSCO has access to adequate infrastructure in terms of National Control laboratories to evaluate the quality of drugs before their final release in the market. The National Institute of Biologicals (NIB), is a notified Central Drug Laboratory for the Quality evaluation of a variety of biologicals whose primary statutory function is to verify the test results of manufacturers – indigenous or importers by way of testing them as per Indian Pharmacopoeia or relevant pharmacopoeia or international norms. This not only helps NRA to evaluate the trend in the quality of biologicals entering the market but also to formulate ways of ensuring the quality of such products before they entered the market. Participating in various international/national external quality assurance assessment schemes/proficiency testing, collaborating on the development of international reference standards for biotherapeutics, and validating studies of test methods meant for quality evaluation of biologicals strengthens the laboratory's testing performance. An independent quality management system (QMS) should support quality control activities with its essential components like the use of validated test procedures; written procedures; knowledgeable, trained, and qualified personnel; management of records and documentation; identification and retention of samples (when appropriate); internal and external audit systems; and oversight procedures.

5.3 STATUTORY REQUIREMENTS FOR QUALITY CONTROL REGULATION OF DIAGNOSTICS

The Medical Device Rules, 2017 is the main piece of legislation in India that governs the production, authorization, import, export, and marketing of medical equipment (MDR-2017). The Drugs and Cosmetics Act of 1940 served as the legal framework for the Medical Device Rules (MDR). The CDSCO at the federal level and the State Licensing Authorities (SLAs) at the state level are responsible for enforcing the D&C Act (including the MDR). The risk-based classification of medical devices was introduced by the Medical Device Rules, 2017. The classification of medical devices is as follows:

Risk Criteria	Risk Class
Low	Class A
Low Moderate	Class B
Moderate High	Class C

Under the said rules, the import of all classes of medical devices as well as the manufacturing of Class C & D medical devices is regulated by CDSCO, while the manufacturing of Class A & B medical devices is regulated by the concerned State Licensing Authorities (SLA) appointed by the State Governments. However, the sale and distribution of all classes of medical devices are regulated by the SLAs.

5.4   ROLE OF QUALITY CONTROL IN CLINICAL LABORATORY

5.4.1   IMPORTANCE OF QUALITY CONTROL IN DIAGNOSTICS

Laboratory diagnosis can be a challenging process that involves, clinical evaluation, microbiological or molecular investigation, or blood banking tests among other aspects of the diagnostic laboratory. One of the most significant effects of quality control (QC) on laboratory testing is that it ensures the accuracy and precision of patient sample results. Both managing overall quality and fulfilling proficiency test criteria depend on the reliability of quality control samples. QC problems, such as reagent matrix effects and calibration misalignment of testing function, must be addressed to identify possible inaccuracies with patient findings. It is crucial to maintain accurate and regular assessments of laboratory sample testing through quality control to ensure that patient testing is carried out properly and that it yields reliable results. Before potentially inaccurate patient findings are disclosed, quality control may identify and correct problems in a lab's analytical procedures, if it functions effectively. A laboratory can self-regulate its testing and ensure that the results are accurate and precise by following quality control procedures. Clinical laboratories optimize the whole quality control process by managing documents and implementing a continuous improvement strategy. Validation of precision and accuracy of test results of the patient sample is done by conducting repeated QC testing. Peer testing and alternative monthly analysis of QC trends are additional methods of managing quality control. Clinical laboratories routinely participate in proficiency testing (PT) programs, which are used to assess/verify their testing procedures. To maintain the quality control of patient samples, periodic assessment of QC findings is frequently used. [19]. PT programs are not only great for assessing QC performance, but they may also assist the lab personnel in identifying problems with reagents even when controls and calibrators appear to be functioning well. The accuracy of sample testing is ensured by the detection of QC deviations from specified ranges on a daily basis, but longer-term assessments are more advantageous for identifying patterns and biases in tests that could be overlooked on a daily basis. The Levey-Jennings chart can also be used to employ patients' samples to serve as controls in the absence of quality control samples [20]. Following the patient findings' running averages, laboratory personnel can spot drift or analyze operational issues that quality control testing fails to detect. For laboratory managers dealing with issues relating to QC materials and recall issues are regular tasks.

Before releasing the results of the patients, the laboratory performs quality control (QC) to identify and minimize mistakes in the analytical stage of the testing system. It takes dedication towards all the stages of the testing system viz. preanalytical, analytical, and post-analytical phases to provide high-quality laboratory results. Preanalytical phase encompasses those variables/elements that might impact laboratory results before the sample is handled in the clinical laboratory. Post-analytical variables are those that have an impact on the outcomes following the analytical phase. Implementing both internal quality control (IQC) and external quality control (EQC) also referred to as proficiency testing (PT), is a component of quality control. While the laboratory conducts daily internal quality control using controls with known values, external quality control involves the laboratory's involvement in an external quality evaluation scheme that serves as a test of competency. Statistical as well as graphical techniques facilitate the interpretation of quality control data. Quality control data is most frequently illustrated with the help of quality control (QC) charts including Levey-Jennings (LJ) charts and Westgard rules. In identifying trends or shifts from the average target value, both are helpful. A key strategy for enhancing the efficiency of a laboratory's quality management system is corrective and preventive action (CAPA). Seamless completion of the root-cause analysis of any issue or deviation can be done by using CAPA in the lab. New management techniques have been developed to control the quality and appropriateness of results. The laboratories have been enabled to continuously enhance their quality control through the use of internal quality control (IQC) and external quality control (EQC). Accreditation and active participation in external quality assessment (EQA) are crucial steps toward assuring accurate, precise, and reliable laboratory test results [21].

5.4.2 QUALITY MANAGEMENT SYSTEM (QMS)

As vital as it is in any other institution, quality is crucial in industries. It can be summed up as the timeliness, correctness, and dependability of reported test results. In industries, quality management systems guarantee the dependability of all processes. The QMS in industries demands quality in all processes, including the environment, quality procedures, record keeping, human resources, reagents, equipment, and instruments. One should be aware that a quality management system used in a laboratory differs from one used electronically (eQMS). An eQMS can help a QMS in a lab setting with record keeping, corrective action (CA) management, document control, and other things.

5.4.2.1 Quality Control and Quality Assurance

Quality control is defined by ISO as part of the quality management requirements mandatory to fulfil accreditation. Some accrediting organizations use the information in ISO 15189 to guide the inspection and accreditation process. The ISO standard provides guidance on implementing regulatory requirements. The component of quality management known as quality assurance is concerned with fostering trust that the standards for quality will be met. A quality management system's implementation is a practical technique to guarantee that the industry or the laboratory's QC and QA objectives are met and upheld.

The laboratory/biological industry quality management systems' 12 pillars: the foundation of a quality management system is comprised of the quality system basics. For the QMS to guarantee accurate, dependable, and speedy findings, all 12 requirements must be met. Although implementing a QMS can help maintain a high-quality laboratory or work place that can identify errors and stop them from happening again, it cannot additionally provide an error-free work flow.

Organization: the management must promote the QMS and find strategies to make personnel aware of its significance.

The following key organizational elements are listed under this quality principle:

- Leadership: the willingness of leaders to participate in the implementation process through team development, motivating techniques, and communication abilities.
- Structure: an organizational chart is required to define the organization's structure properly.
- Planning: a strategy for skill development should be established
- Implementation: management must handle any difficulties with the QMS.
- Monitoring: systems for monitoring make sure that QMS designs adhere to standards. Additionally, it is essential for ongoing development.
- Personnel: in a laboratory/workplace, they are in charge of implementing and upholding the QMS. The workplace director is in charge of creating accurate job descriptions and hiring qualified personnel. He or she should also be in charge of making sure they receive ongoing education and keep up with emerging trends and technologies.

Employees must go through a performance evaluation, which will include a thorough assessment of factors like policy adherence, safety protocol compliance, communication abilities, punctuality, and behavior.

- Equipment: it is crucial to have equipment that is in good working order because it will improve output, confidence, and dependability. Additionally, it extends service life and reduces repair expenses. Installation, calibration, maintenance, troubleshooting, and validation are all steps that can be taken to ensure effective equipment management.
- Purchasing and inventory: this section outlines the contracts the laboratory has with clients and outside vendors to guarantee that demands for essential supplies and services are routinely met. The availability of inventory when needed and the efficiency and cost-effectiveness of operations are both guaranteed by proper purchasing and inventory rules.
- Process control: it covers actions taken to ensure that requirements are met and that resources are used effectively, both directly and indirectly related to the workflow of the laboratory. Sample management is one of the procedures essential to laboratory performance. The sample must be carefully preserved under the advised conditions as soon as it is collected to avoid deterioration.
- Information management: offers instructions for controlling the information created and entered into laboratory record-keeping systems, including patient demographics, test results, reports, and interpretations.
- Records and documents: all necessary data must be accessible and readily available. They must be updated, and information must be recorded using specified forms and formats.
- Occurrence management: occurrences must be looked into for the underlying causes when they are discovered. Future occurrences are avoided by doing this. By adopting the proper corrective and preventive actions after an incident is discovered, it can be fixed (CAPAs).
- Assessment: assessment is a crucial quality concept that assesses every QMS function and shows that it complies with legal and customer criteria. Instead of assessments, ISO employs audits.
- Process improvement: in accordance with ISO 15189, a process should be continually improved by identifying deficiencies, developing an improvement plan, putting it into practice, evaluating its success, and making adjustments.
- Customer service: the clients (patients, physicians, and public health organizations) must be satisfied, and the head is in charge of monitoring this. Surveys, indicators, and audits are just a few of the several methods that can be used to gauge satisfaction.
- Facilities and safety: the head is in charge of maintaining safety and quality. He or she must actively take part in design, evaluate all potential dangers, and offer suggestions for creating a secure lab.

The requirements for quality management that must be met in order to receive accreditation include quality control. Another component of quality management, quality assurance, is to give customers confidence that the quality standards will be met. Implementing a quality management system is the most efficient way to guarantee that the quality control and quality assurance objectives are accomplished and maintained. Although implementing a quality management system does not ensure an industry/laboratory is error-free, it does assist in identifying potential faults and preventing them from happening again. Contrarily, biological industries that do not use a quality management system ensure that mistakes will not be caught.

Three stages make up the cyclical process of laboratory/biological testing: preanalytical, analytical, and post-analytical. QMS is a coordinated way to manage laboratory operations to guarantee precise, dependable, and timely results for clinical and public health applications [22].

A standard operating procedure (SOP) is a document that details routinely occurring operations to guarantee that they are performed accurately (quality) and consistently (consistency). Even when there are staff changes, it makes sure businesses stay consistent and do not take unneeded safety risks. The foundation of regulatory compliance operations is it. The first violation of compliance is "failure to follow written directions," while the second violation is "absence of recorded instructions."

To ensure quality, it is important to address every aspect of the biological industries operation, including its organizational structure, the SOPs used for testing, good laboratory practices (GLPs), qualified and competent staff, good equipment, standard reagents, quality control procedures, record inventory, and effective communication. In order to ensure the accuracy and reliability of testing, a variety of procedures and processes are included in the biological industry. A flaw in any component of the system could produce fictitious and incorrect results. Indian biological industry quality management seeks to guarantee findings that are precise, consistent, and traceable; trained, competent, and safe employees; defined processes and procedures; records that are kept; satisfied clients; and an ever-improving system.

5.4.2.2 Elements of Quality Management System

It is very important to adopt high-quality standards in all operations, testing procedures, and reporting in any biological industry. A quality management system ensures that every product manufactured and marketed must comply with the required standards. To maintain quality, well-defined and documented procedures and systems should be in place, which are strictly complied with. There are 12 quality system basics in the QMS model, and each one must be handled to ensure correctness and dependability along the workflow route in a way that is appropriate for the laboratory [23].

5.4.2.3 Accreditation and Certification

The recognition of the biological industries competence and quality is called accreditation. When a QMS is in place and it complies with the quality standard, it is said to be successful. Any biological industry must submit to an evaluation body by a notified independent accreditation authority in order to apply for accreditation. This assessment is used to establish whether the QMS is actually operating as planned and whether the laboratory complies with the quality standard. An essential element in the QMS' ongoing progress is accreditation. The industries evaluate their performance to determine whether it is comparable to a benchmark, which enables them to revise their policies or methods for ongoing improvement. Assessments, including those for accreditation, certification, or licensure, can be carried out in a variety of methods. Because accreditation also includes a competency assessment, it gives users of the biological industry a higher level of assurance that the testing is correct and dependable.

Many industries employ the International Standardization Organization (ISO) certification, which is a documented guarantee from an independent organization that a product, method, or service complies with certain requirements [23]. Accreditation is a higher level of quality than certification since it is a formal declaration by an authoritative organization that a person or institution is qualified or able to carry out a given duty. Representatives from an accreditation authority visit the lab to verify that it complies with standards, rules, policies, procedures, and regulations as well as to make sure the personnel is competently and correctly carrying out their responsibilities and obligations. While the ISO 15189 standard is applicable to clinical laboratories/industries, the ISO/IEC 17025 standard is used to accredit testing or calibration laboratories/industries. The decision between certification and accreditation is based on the needs of regulatory agencies, incoming client requests, or planned laboratory growth. An organization gains from accreditation in a number of ways. It makes it easier for the organization to create and maintain a successful quality system. The laboratory/biological industry produces the results and gains faith in the accuracy and dependability of the findings. Customers are reassured of appropriate laboratory practices, which increases their willingness to use the services. The decision-makers can rely on the test results since they are trustworthy. It gives the laboratory national and international validation of its technical proficiency and so ensures global equivalency. By producing findings that are accurate the first time and every time, it automatically lowers the operational expenses of the industry/laboratories as all regulatory requirements for all the procedures involved in testing are met, starting with the purchase of materials and reagents. Increased business and governmental usage and acceptance of results from accredited laboratories/biological industries, including results from industries/laboratories in other nations, is the ultimate goal of accreditation. The free-trade principle of "product tested once, approved everywhere" can be achieved in this fashion. In other words, certification increases client confidence by formally recognizing the competence of accreditation bodies, hence eliminating the need for additional testing as a technical trade barrier.

5.4.2.4 Implementation of the Laboratory Quality Management System

A pandemic outbreak necessitates rapid diagnosis and precise results reporting. However, it is advisable to put into practice a QMS's practical suggestions in order to improve the running of the biological industry and produce accurate results. For instance, while setting up any laboratory related to biological/diagnostic/virology laboratory, the WHO recommends three essential components: (a) physical infrastructure; (b) human resources; and (c) equipment and supplies [23].

Safety programs for other catastrophes, including fires, earthquakes, power outages, spills, and medical emergencies, should also be in place, in addition to adhering to the prescribed biosafety procedures.

A routine for monitoring the environmental conditions, including the ambient temperature, should also be established.

Equipment should constantly be maintained according to a preventative maintenance schedule. Every piece of equipment should have a troubleshooting process in place. It is essential to guarantee that everyone using the equipment has undergone the necessary training, is knowledgeable about how to use it efficiently, and is capable of performing the necessary routine maintenance procedures.

Consideration must be given to the following factors for efficient equipment management:

- Installation: the equipment should be installed properly to enable accessibility, efficient workflow, and sequential use. Prior to use, the new equipment must have its performance validated. Equipment must also be calibrated on a regular basis.
- Regular maintenance: an SOP for the upkeep and repair of equipment should exist. Both internal preventative maintenance and vendor-provided maintenance/repair are crucial. Before beginning any repair work, the working area and equipment need to be properly decontaminated.
- Equipment inventory: a system for keeping track of equipment is helpful. Each piece of equipment used to conduct examinations should have a record kept of it.

To implement the QMS in an effective way, the activities are grouped into four implementation phases, where each phase has a specific focus [24]. The four phases for implementation of quality management include the following:

- Phase 1: making sure that the working area's main process functions correctly and safely
- Phase 2: quality control and assurance and establishing traceability
- Phase 3: assuring effective management, leadership, and organization
- Phase 4: developing a continual improvement system and becoming ready for accreditation

The overall quality of biological industry procedures is enhanced by the introduction of QMS. The provision of prompt and accurate care for patients is made possible by the major reduction of errors and the ongoing improvement of quality, efficiency, and outcomes. The attainment of quality standards in the Indian biological industry is the result of the QMS's implementation, which is done so in a methodical, step-by-step manner while addressing all quality essentials. However, extensive follow-up, monitoring, and continued documentation are necessary to ensure the long-term success of implementing QMS programs.

5.5 CONCLUSION

By providing high-quality medications in large quantities, the Indian pharmaceutical and biological industry has solidified its position in the global generics market. The industry has transformed itself into a dependable, high-quality, and economical worldwide drug supplier through advancements in processes and formulations. The sector has dominated the market share in developed economies all over the world by lowering the cost of vital medications and increasing their accessibility. To attain the desired levels of CAGR, however, joint efforts from all stakeholders, including Indian pharmaceutical businesses, the government, and regulatory bodies, are required. To promote this innovation-led growth, government involvement in the form of investments, policy support, and regulatory interventions is essential and praiseworthy. The impact can be accelerated by considering the following tactical elements.

- Using digital technology, to hasten and enhance the healthcare infrastructure.
- Establish a stable and benevolent regulatory setting so that businesses can plan its investments.
- Foster innovation by building a research ecosystem, and establish India as a center of the life sciences.
- Increase the talent pool's capabilities to handle complex technology.
- Consolidate and broaden global presence while working with international regulatory organizations to create global policies, rules, and regulations.

5.6 CASE STUDIES

Case Study 1: Vaccine Manufacturing in India

Several large government-backed companies have contributed significantly to the production of various vaccines, making India one of the world's leading vaccine producers. In terms of doses produced, the Serum Institute of India (SII) is the largest vaccine factory in the world. Thanks to the company's pivotal role in the COVID-19 pandemic, the world now has access to affordable and accessible vaccines.

SII has developed a novel coronavirus vaccine, Oxford AstraZeneca, known as Covishield in India during the pandemic. Through licensing agreements and knowledge transfer, SII has rapidly expanded production to meet domestic and international demand.

As shown in this case study, Indian companies like SII have demonstrated their technological prowess and manufacturing capabilities in the production of life-saving biologics, forming strategic partnerships to effectively address global health challenges.

Case Study 2: Biopharmaceutical Export Growth
Indian biopharmaceutical companies have expanded their presence in the global market in recent years.

Bangalore-based biopharmaceutical company Biocon Limited provides a striking example. Biocon is a leader in the development and export of high-quality biologics and biosimilars to various countries. The company's lead drug, insulin glargine, became the first Indian-made biosimilars to be approved in Europe. The company has also established itself in emerging markets by providing cost-effective, life-saving biologics for chronic diseases, such as diabetes and cancer.

This case study explores how an Indian biopharmaceutical company embraced innovation, adhered to stringent quality standards and negotiated a challenging regulatory process to achieve global prestige and positive impact on healthcare systems around the world.

Case Study 3: Regulating Biologicals in India
Management of biologics is critical to ensuring patient safety and product efficacy. India's Central Drug Standards Control Organization (CDSCO) is responsible for the regulation of biologics and pharmaceuticals. The launch process for Bharat Biotech's Covaxin, a locally manufactured COVID-19 vaccine, is a case study worth considering.

Regulatory authorities are scrutinizing Covaxin to ensure compliance with safety, efficacy, and quality requirements. During the pandemic, the vaccine was approved for emergency use and then reviewed for full approval.

This case study demonstrates how Indian regulators can help maintain a vibrant biologics ecosystem by balancing the need for emergency immediacy while ensuring product quality and patient safety.

These case studies provide insight into a wide range of Indian companies and their role in biologics production, export, and regulation. These demonstrate India's potential as a leading player in the global biopharmaceutical sector and contribute to advances in medicine and public health on a global scale.

Case Study 4: Biotechnology Advancements in the Indian Pharmaceutical Industry
In recent years, the Indian pharmaceutical sector has grown into a global player, with a particular focus on biological and biotechnology-based products. An interesting case study concerns the development and manufacturing of biosimilar pharmaceuticals in India.

In this example, an Indian pharmaceutical company recognized the growing global market for biosimilars and sought to capitalize on it. They have invested strategically in research and development and built state-of-the-art biotechnology facilities to produce high-quality biosimilars. They have also tapped India's vast scientific expertise by collaborating with leading academic and research institutes.

Through careful development and strict quality control, the company has obtained regulatory approvals for a range of biosimilar products, including monoclonal antibodies and recombinant proteins. These biosimilars not only fill an unmet medical need, but also provide a cheaper alternative to expensive original biologics and make medicine more accessible to individuals.

This case study shows how Indian pharmaceutical companies are leveraging biotechnology and new approaches to compete in the global market, contributing significantly to the growth of the country's biopharmaceutical sector.

Case Study 5: Vaccine Manufacturing during a Pandemic
During the COVID-19 pandemic, the global demand for vaccines increased dramatically, placing a heavy burden on vaccine manufacturers worldwide. Several Indian companies have responded by playing a key role in the production of COVID-19 vaccines.

An Indian biopharmaceutical company has teamed up with a global vaccine manufacturer to rapidly transform its manufacturing facility to produce a COVID-19 vaccine. Despite extraordinary hurdles, such as scaling up production, maintaining strict quality control, and negotiating a complex regulatory process, the company has successfully produced millions of doses of the vaccine, making a significant contribution to global immunization efforts bottom.

This case study demonstrates the adaptability and resilience of Indian biopharmaceutical companies in crisis, demonstrating the company's ability to rapidly respond to public health disasters and contribute to global vaccine availability.

These case studies highlight the significant progress made by Indian companies in the fields of biotechnology and biology. They demonstrate how Indian companies have leveraged technology upgrades, innovation, and strategic partnerships to establish themselves as major players in the global biopharmaceutical business. Given India's favorable environment for biotechnology development, India's contributions in this area are likely to have long-term implications not only for human health, but beyond as well.

Case Study 6: Indian Biotechnology Industry's Growth Trajectory
Background
Over the final two decades, the Indian biotechnology industry has developed drastically, much appreciated to a strong administrative system, an endless pool of talented researchers and engineers, and a solid accentuation on investigate and improvement. The biopharmaceutical segment, which deals with biological products, such as immunizations, therapeutic proteins, and monoclonal antibodies, has seen colossal development as a result of this extension.

Case study: within the early 2000s, an Indian biotech firm arranged to go into biopharmaceutical advancement and manufacture. They perceived the worldwide biologics market's gigantic potential and found chances to meet both domestic and worldwide request.

Challenges: the company faced many obstacles when entering the biopharmaceutical market. To begin with, they must contribute significantly in the background, equipment, and skills to build state-of-the-art bioprocessing offices and learn about research facilities. At one point, they had to navigate complex administrative channels, including the strict rules of global regulators, such as the Food and Drug Administration (FDA) and the European Medicines Agency (EMA).

Solutions: to overcome these problems, the company has partnered with leading global biotech companies to transfer technology and know-how. This strategic alliance allows them to accelerate the learning and implementation of best practices in bioremediation and quality control. In addition, they have hired proficient scientists and management experts from world-renowned biopharmaceutical companies to oversee their R&D activities.

Outcomes: as part of its strategic strategy, the company has successfully built a pipeline of high-value biological products, including biosimilars and innovative biologics. The company's products have been approved by numerous regulatory bodies, allowing it to enter the international market. In addition, through strict quality control, we have a reputation for reliability and safety, and we are strengthening our international competitiveness.

Impact: the success of this Indian biotech company has not only boosted the Indian biopharmaceutical sector but also contributed to the country's status as a hotspot for biotech innovation. Making biopharmaceuticals more affordable and accessible not only meets local health needs, but exporting low-cost biopharmaceuticals to developing countries is also important in solving global health problems.

REFERENCES

1. USFDA, Healthcare Providers (Biologics). [Last accessed 2019 Jan 19]. www. fda. gov/BiologicsBloodVaccines/ResourcesforYou/ HealthcareProviders/default.html .
2. Morrow T, Felcone LH. Defining the difference: what makes biologics unique. Biotechnology Healthcare 2004;1:24–9.
3. Wijesinghe H, Seneviratne SL, Galappatthy P, Wijayaratne L. Biologics: a new weapon in the war against autoimmune joint disease. Journal of the Ceylon College of Physicians 2010;41:76–82.
4. Park SH, Aniwan S, Loftus EV., Jr Advances in the use of biologics and other novel drugs for managing inflammatory bowel disease. Current Opinion in Pharmacology. 2017;37:65–71.
5. Blackstone EA, Joseph PF. The economics of biosimilars. American Health and Drug Benefits. 2013;6:469–78.
6. Hofmarcher T, Jönsson B, Wilking N. Access to high-quality oncology care across Europe. IHE Report 2014: 2, IHE: Lund. [Last accessed on 2018 July 2].
7. EUROPEAN MEDICINES AGENCY, Biosimilarmedicnes: Overview. [Last accesses on 2018 June 20]. www.ema.europa.eu/en/human-regulatory/ overview/ biosimilar-medicines.

8. Owens DR, Landgraf W, Schmidt A, Bretzel RG, Kuhlmann MK. The emergence of biosimilar insulin preparations—a cause for concern? Diabetes Technology & Therapeutics. 2012;14:989–96.

9. Ghosh PK. Similar biologics: global opportunities and issues. Journal of Pharmacy & Pharmaceutical Sciences 2017;19:552–96.

10. Sullivan T. 2017 Biosimilar Update, Policy and Medicine. [Last accessed on 2018 Jan 2]. www.policymed.com/2017/02/2017-biosimilar-update.

11. Guidelines on Similar Biologic: Regulatory Requirements for Marketing Authorization in India. [Last accessed on January 2019 17]. www.cdsco.nic.in.

12. GUIDELINE ON SIMILAR BIOLOGICS: Regulatory Requirements for Marketing Authorization in India. 2016. [Last accessed on 2018 June 22]. www.dbtindia.nic.in/wp-content/uploads/10.- Guidelines-on-Similar-Biologics-2016.pdf.

13. Brennan Z India Releases New Biosimilars Guidance, Regulatory Focus. [Last accessed on 2018 June 23]. www.raps.org/regulatoryfocus% E2%84%A2/news-articles/2016/3/India-releases-newbiosimilars- guidance.

14. Meher BR, Balan S, Mohanty RR, Jena M, Das S. Biosimilars in India; current status and future perspectives. Journal of Pharmacy and Bioallied Sciences 2019 Jan–Mar;11(1):12–15. doi: 10.4103/jpbs.JPBS_167_18. PMID: 30906134; PMCID: PMC6394151.

15. Chan JCN, Chan ATC. Biologics and biosimilars: what, why and how? ESMO Open. 2017 Mar 24; 2(1):e000180. doi: 10.1136/esmoopen-2017-000180. PMCID: PMC5519784.

16. www.biosimilardevelopment.com/doc/the-opportunities-challenges-of-india-s-biologics-market-0001.

17. www.biosimilardevelopment.com/doc/the-opportunities-challenges-of-india-s-biologics-market-0001.

18. https://morulaa.com/cdsco/regulation-of-biologics-in-india-2/-.

19. Karkalousos P, Evangelopoulos A. Quality control in clinical laboratories. Applications and experiences of quality control, Prof. OgnyanIvanov (Ed.). 2011; ISBN: 978-953-307-236-4, In Tech.

20. Crellin M, Cavagnara M, Arneson W (2007). Quality assessment. In: Ameson W, Brickell J editors, Clinical Chemistry: A Laboratory Perspective. Philadelphia: F.A. Davis; 2007. p. 582.

21. Raj A. A review on corrective and preventive action (CAPA). African Journal of Pharmacy and Pharmacology 2016;10:1–6.

22. Clinical and Laboratory Standards Institute. QMS01: QMS – A Model for Laboratory Services CLSI. [Last accessed on 2020 Oct 13]. Available from https://clsi. Org/standards/products/quality-management-systems/documents/ qms01/.

23. WHO. Laboratory Quality Management System: Handbook. [Last accessed on 2020 Oct 13]. Available from www.who.int/ihr/publications/lqms/en/.

24. WHO. Laboratory Quality Management System (LQMS) Training Toolkit. [Last accessed on 2020 Oct 13]. Available from www.who.int/ihr/training/laboratory_quality/introduction/en/.

6 Animal-Based Testing Methods and Their Alternatives in Quality Control Evaluation of Biologicals

Anoop Kumar
National Institute of Biologicals, Ministry of Health and Family Welfare, Government of India, A-32, Sector-62, Noida – 201309, India

6.1 BACKGROUND

Biologicals are the class of medicine derived from living organisms like bacteria or yeast, or plant or animal cells. It includes vaccines, monoclonal antibodies, growth factors, and human blood/plasma-derived products [1]. The testing and regulation of biological products are different due to their nature and production methods. Therefore, it is very essential to ensure the efficacy, safety, and quality of the biologicals by testing at each step. The quality control evaluation of biologicals is an important aspect of the safety, and effectiveness of the product that involves in vitro, in vivo, and physiochemical processes. The use of laboratory animals is essential for the quality evaluation of biologicals to evaluate their potency, toxicity, and pyrogenicity, which has to be used in humans and animals (Figure 6.1).

In vivo tests (within living organisms), such as the rabbit pyrogen test, abnormal toxicity test, virus inactivation test, evaluation of skin reactions, and potency assays, enable the testing of biological entities in living organisms rather than in human tissue or dead organisms. Prior to administering the product to humans or the species of animal, it is intended for, it may be tested on animals first before being administered to larger populations. It may also be tested on animals before marketing approval, or to guarantee quality during production [2].

India has emerged as one of the leading providers of biologicals to the world market for similar biologics. Regulation of the biologicals for the manufacturing, import, and export of genetically engineered organisms or cell storage, are under

DOI: 10.1201/9781032697444-6

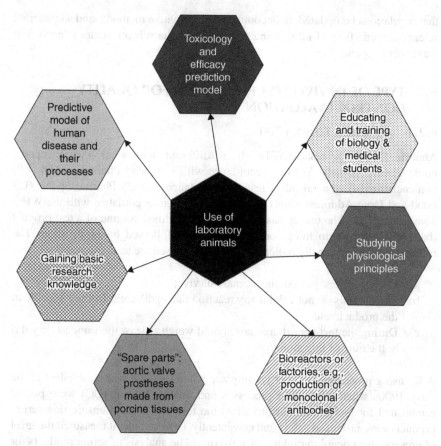

FIGURE 6.1 Use of laboratory animals.

the Drug and Cosmetic Act 1940 and The Drugs and Cosmetic Rules 1945. In India, regulation of biologicals, their approval for preclinical and clinical trials, new drug application (NDA), and their import/export are being taken care of by governing bodies, such as the Central Drugs Standard Control Organization (CDSCO) and the Drugs Controller General of India (DCGI).

In terms of fundamental research, non-clinical testing, and quality control of biological has the highest percentage of animal trials that hurt and distress them. As alternatives to animal testing are being developed, quality control evaluation of biologicals is experiencing substantial momentum. Additionally, there are technical developments in the realm of analytical methods and their application.

As a result, the 3Rs, i.e., replacement, refinement, and reduction, can be employed in specific animal-based tests, and the consistency methodology can be applied as a quality strategy [3]. The scientific progress alone, however, will not guarantee the acceptance of the 3Rs by all stakeholders, worldwide. It is imperative that regulations be updated, to accommodate alternative methods, and a concerted science-driven effort of influencing and including the subject matter is needed to make this happen.

6.2 TYPE OF IN VIVO TEST PERFORMED FOR QUALITY CONTROL EVALUATION

6.2.1 ABNORMAL TOXICITY TEST

Abnormal toxicity tests (ATTs) have different names in Pharmacopoeia nomenclature, namely ATTs in accordance with European Pharmacopoeia (EP) nomenclature [4], general safety tests in accordance with US Pharmacopoeia (US Food and Drug Administration), or innocuity tests in accordance with the WHO nomenclature [1] The test consists of injecting a defined volume of a test product (batch) at a time into mice and/or guinea pigs, followed by observation. The following criteria typically indicate that a batch passed the test:

a. During the test period, the animals survive;
b. The animals do not exhibit any reaction that is different from or specific to the product; and
c. During the test period, animals should weigh at least the same as they did at the time of injection.

A licensing procedure was not yet in place when the ATT was established in the early 1900s when production processes and quality control (QC) were poorly established for biologicals. At this time, the test was used to ensure that serum products were produced safely and consistently. For example, it measured the level of preservative phenol in diphtheria antiserum. The analysis of serum products for phenol was insufficient due to the lack of analytical techniques. The detection of toxic levels of phenol was therefore carried out using mice, as they are a susceptible species. As a biological indicator for tetanus toxin, guinea pigs were introduced around 1900 as a test for antiserum formulations [5].

6.2.2 RABBIT PYROGEN TEST

Rabbit pyrogen testing (RPT) is a qualitative technique used to determine whether parenteral preparations contain contaminating (fever-causing) pyrogens by measuring the temperature changes of rabbits after giving a test sample. In 1912, Hort and Penfold first used it to investigate the causes of fever caused by injectables in patients [6]. In both, National Control Laboratories (NCLs) and manufacturers, this method is used to determine pyrogen content.

Pyrogen is a substance that induces a fever, such as lipopolysaccharides (LPS) produced by Gram-negative bacteria (endotoxins). Pyrogens pose a considerable hazard to human health when they are used in health products [7, 8]. The pyrogens contaminating the test were found to be of bacterial origin in the 1920s by Seibert [9]. This test gained popularity during the Second World War due to the high demand for intravenous solutions. The pharmacopoeia methods have been refined over the years, and rabbit screening has been added before use to decrease the figure of false positives [10]. In many cases, the bacterial endotoxin test (BET) has replaced the RPT due to its scientific and ethical shortcomings. RPT is considered an "industry standard" because it has been an established pharmacopoeia method for detecting non-endotoxin pyrogens (NEPS) for many years.

When pyrogenic contaminants are present in the parenteral (mainly intravenous), they can cause a fatal systemic immune response in the patient. There can be symptoms ranging from fever to septic shock-like symptoms. In RPT, three rabbits are administered with pyrogen intravenously for 180 minutes, while their body temperature is monitored. Temperature increases (fever) must be within defined temperature ranges [11] in order to fulfil the drug's requirements. While EP, USP, and JP have different setups, they all generate the same level of safety [12]. As its design implies, it is a qualitative (pass/fail) safety test for drugs that are typically non-pyrogenic.

6.2.3 POTENCY

It is the ability of a biological to exert the desired effect in patients in vivo that defines its potency. Biologicals' potency is equivalent to pharmaceutical strength [13]. Strength is typically determined by the amount of active ingredients in pharmaceutical products. It is assumed that the product will be potent if it contains the appropriate amount of active ingredients.

In vivo animal testing should be accompanied under appropriate conditions after appropriate validation for any potency assay based on animals. It may be worthwhile to consider some principles outlined in current guidelines for biological tests of prophylactic vaccines and their statistical analysis (e.g., Ph. Eur. 2.7 & 5.3.6).

6.3 ADVANTAGES AND LIMITATIONS OF ANIMAL-BASED TESTING

Often, an animal model is used to mimic how human bodies respond to diseases and medications. Medical technology has led to an increase in the number of animals used in research. All over the world, millions of animals are used for experimental purposes every year. Research using animals in the UK was estimated at 3.71 million in 2011 [14].

Scientific merit has been lost, and the ATT has neither been proven, reproducible, nor reliable, nor is it appropriate for its intended purpose. The ATT is not considered suitable as a QC release test, since it does not provide explicit and reproducible results that might enable batch release decisions.

6.3.1 ADVANTAGES OF ANIMAL-BASED RABBIT PYROGEN TEST

- In the pyrogen test, rabbits were used since they are similar to humans when it comes to their sensitivity to endotoxins [15].
- The RPT is designed to mimic the administration of parenteral drugs through intravenous (IV) routes of administration, which is the same route prescribed in the pharmacopoeia.
- Sensitivity to pyrogens is much greater when delivered IV, an essential consideration when modeling a response to endotoxin.

6.3.2 LIMITATION OF ANIMAL-BASED RABBIT PYROGEN TEST

- If numerous other compounds, both endogenous and exogenous, are suspected of triggering the increase in the rabbits' temperature, this could be a noteworthy limiting factor in exploiting this test to conclude endotoxins in a sample.
- Although it is improbable that this test will result in a false positive due to endogenous substances due to the large number of subjects tested, it is very common to see incorrect results when the samples are found to be contaminated with a virus, fungus, or any other type of substance that could cause fever in all of the animals tested [16].
- It has the disadvantage of only providing a qualitative response, and cannot quantify the number of endotoxins in a sample.
- Blood plasma, e.g., contains endotoxins that are in an inactive state when injected, but become toxic over time and ultimately cause fevers due to metabolic processes that plasma goes through in the body.
- It is not uncommon for the pyrogen method to yield a false-negative result in rabbits.

6.3.3 ADVANTAGES OF ANIMAL-BASED POTENCY ASSAYS

- The mechanism of therapeutic efficacy may accurately reflect the efficacy of the treatment
- In a single assay, multiple functional domains can be assessed
- Suitable cell lines may not be present

6.3.4 LIMITATION OF ANIMAL-BASED POTENCY ASSAYS

- Animal ethical issues and high costs associated with animal housing and husbandry
- Test durations can be long, increasing the time it takes for batches to be released
- Despite rigorous protocols, animal studies within species do not always demonstrate reproducibility
- High rate of invalidation

- Challenging to standardize
- Challenging to transfer to new testing sites

6.4 ALTERNATIVE METHODS FOR ANIMAL-BASED TESTING

Substitute to animal testing were suggested to overcome certain shortcomings allied with animal experiments and evade unethical measures. A policy of 3Rs is being implemented, which stances for the reduction, refinement, and replacement of laboratory animals [17]. A three-step strategy is implemented aimed at reducing, refining, and replacing animal use in laboratories (Figure 6.2).

Compared to animal testing, alternative methods for evaluating quality are more resilient, have lower interassay variability, are more precise, and can be completed in a shorter period of time. The regulatory agencies are thus required to conduct specific tests on biologicals to ensure their safety, purity, efficacy, and identity. Safety and efficacy testing is necessary for batch releases of biologicals, and this necessitates the use of a large number of animals, but in vitro testing may be a more feasible alternative (non-animal methods). The international legislation and standards relating to animal welfare and safety have been reaffirmed to help vaccine manufacturers and laboratories to ensure the safety and effectiveness of their biologicals. Due to this, it is imperative to develop, validate, and implement new in vitro procedures as quickly as feasible. Furthermore, when it comes to batch testing, these techniques may be ethical, safer time, and money-saving.

6.4.1 ALTERNATIVE METHODS ABNORMAL TOXICITY TESTS (ATTs)

The ATT's ability to identify potentially dangerous batches is scientifically questionable; the test is inconsistent, non-reproducible, and non-specific. Under GMP, where suitable procedures using cutting-edge approaches for product control and release are in place, the ATT is not considered to offer any useful information. Over 80 product monographs of the EP have been amended to eliminate the ATT as part of recent amendments and removed it from EP supplement 9.6 (effective January 1, 2019). In 2015, the U.S.21 CFR for biologicals was amended so that the

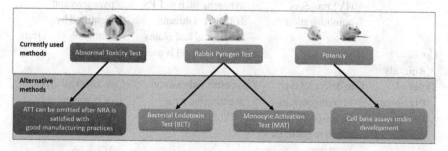

FIGURE 6.2 Alternatives to animal-based testing in evaluating the quality of biologicals.

General Safety Test (GST) was revoked. In harmony with the amendment, certain safety tests are required only for certain products if they are identified in an approved Biologics License Application (BLA) that presents specific safety concerns. On a regulatory level, these changes demonstrate commitment to the 3Rs:

- Older requirements need to be amended
- The ability to accept and use new technology as it develops
- Test capabilities that are evolving and new must be accepted

6.4.2 ALTERNATIVE METHODS TO RABBIT PYROGEN TEST

Presently there are few tests defined in Pharmacopeia as an alternative to RPT that detects the majority of the pyrogens (Table 6.1) and they are as follows:

- The BET, i.e., limulus polyphemus amoebocyte lysate-test (LAL-test), effectively substituted the rabbit pyrogen test for many products
- Monocyte activation test (MAT), identifies pyrogens and endotoxins from Gram-positive bacteria

6.4.2.1 Bacterial Endotoxin Test

In the 1980s, the US pharmacopoeia (USP) introduced the BET, also called limulus amebocyte lysate (LAL), as an alternative to the RPT. This test reduces the use

TABLE 6.1
Comparison of the Available Pyrogen Test Methods

	Rabbit Pyrogen Test	Bacterial Endotoxin Test	Monocyte Activation Test
Principle	Designed to mimic the administration of parenteral drugs through intravenous (IV) routes of administration	A method based on the reaction of the horseshoe crab (Limulus polyphemus) hemolymph with pyrogens such as LPS, 1(3)-β-D- Glucans from fungi and plants	Cytokines and interleukins (IL) are produced by activated monocytes in response to pyrogens and identified by immunological tests.
Use of Animals	High	Low (only Blood is used)	No
Types of Pyrogens Detected	Can detect all type of pyrogen, e.g., Gram-positive and negative bacteria, yeast, etc.	Can detect only Gram-negative bacteria	Can detect all types of pyrogens, e.g., Gram-positive and negative bacteria, yeast, etc.

of animals particularly vertebrates, which in turn decreases variability, improves the sensitivity, and speed of the pyrogen test. It involves an in vitro method based on the reaction of the horseshoe crab (Limulus polyphemus) hemolymph with pyrogens such as LPS, 1(3)-β-D-Glucans from fungi and plants [18–20].

In the last couple of decades, LAL tests have replaced rabbit pyrogen tests for about 80% of the cases. To completely phase out RPT and LAL tests there is a need for human-based in vitro tests. Monocyte activation tests, which are only in vitro approaches, mimic human responses to pyrogens by producing cytokines, were quickly accepted as a viable alternative to rabbit pyrogen tests and were included in EP as a compendial method (2010) and USP as an alternative method (2011).

6.4.2.2 Monocyte Activation Test (MAT)

The MAT identifies pyrogens and endotoxins from Gram-positive bacteria and takes the place of the RPT in terms of detecting pyrogens and endotoxins. In this test, monocytes are activated by pyrogens to produce cytokines and interleukins (IL), and these molecules can be detected by an immunological test (e.g., ELISA). The different types of MAT variants are available based on the following:

- Blood, primary human monocytes (e.g., PBMC), or monocytic cell lines can be used as human monocyte sources
- Readout of immunological endpoint assays, such as IL-6, IL-1β, or TNF-α

Monocyte activation test has been described in the E.P. as a compendial technique for pyrogen detection since January 2010. It has been recommended to replace rabbit pyrogen tests with MAT whenever possible and subsequently product-specific validation [21].

6.5 ISSUES WITH ANIMAL-BASED TESTING

Although there are ethical issues and political pressures surrounding animal testing, there are also significant economic, scientific, and regulatory concerns about their uses in this area.

6.5.1 ECONOMIC ISSUES

From an economic standpoint, in vivo tests are expensive, time-consuming, and labor-intensive [22]. In addition to the high costs associated with animal housing and husbandry, test durations can be long, increasing the time it takes for batches to be released. In order to test vaccine potency, for instance, it can take weeks or months. There is a high likelihood of rejection of product batches that are safe and efficacious based on the high inconsistency of in vivo responses, which can lead to retesting and possible investigations into out-of-specification results, as well as further delays in the release of the product or shortages. When NCLs (accountable for post-approval, premarket batch release testing) fail to collaborate with manufacturers, or if their results differ from those of the manufacturer, can result in further delays and costs. It is well known that animal testing increases the costs and timelines associated with manufacturing products under current Good Manufacturing Practices (cGMP), but it adds little or no value to their quality or safety [3].

6.5.2 SCIENTIFIC ISSUES

In terms of quality control evaluation of a biological batch to be released, there are several important issues that need to be addressed from a scientific perspective, including the inherent variability and poor robustness of many in vivo assays, the relevance of animal responses to human health conditions, and the fact that some tests that are still in use have not been validated in harmony with the strict requirements for quality control. In view of the fact that there are interspecies variances in biological responses, animal batch release testing may not be applicable to human safety and efficacy. Furthermore, animal methods are inherently variable, which makes them insufficient for ensuring consistent quality across batches. Non-animal assays utilizing less variability and more readily transferable protocols would be a better way to support the consistency approach [23] for routine releases of biologicals. Some regulatory authorities already recognize and accept the use of non-animal assays as substitutes for in vivo methods for batch release testing and quality control of biologicals [24]. As an alternative to rabbit pyrogenicity tests, the monocyte activation test has now been incorporated into the European pharmacopoeia, while the CHO cell clustering test for monitoring residual pertussis toxin has been added to the mouse histamine sensitization test [21, 25].

6.5.3 REGULATORY ISSUES

There has been a lack of harmonization of regulations and guidelines regarding the safety, efficacy, and potency testing requirements for biologicals resulting in a hampered adoption of 3R methods related to animal testing for licensure and post-licensure release [24, 26]. National regulatory authorities can have different testing requirements and/or batch approval specifications for the same product from different manufacturers and for similar products released in multiple countries by one manufacturer, for example. Furthermore, different regions have different protocol requirements for the same animal assay. Several factors can influence an assay's result, including the strain of the animal, the housing conditions, the time period, controls, or references.

6.6 ADAPTATION OF 3RS IN QUALITY CONTROL

There is a legal and ethical obligation for the countries, which have signed the Convention of the Council of Europe and, in particular, for the MS of the European

Union. Both, the European Convention for the Protection of Animals Used for Experimental and other scientific purposes, ETS 123 (Council of Europe, 1986) and Directive 86/609/EEC (EEC, 1986) claim that

- "an (animal) experiment shall not be performed if another scientifically satisfactory method of obtaining the result sought, not entailing the use of an animal, is reasonable and practicably available"; (replacement)
- "in a choice between experiments, those which use the minimum number of animals or cause the least pain, suffering, distress, and lasting harm and which are most likely to provide satisfactory results shall be selected"; (reduction and refinement) and
- "all experiments shall be designed to avoid distress and unnecessary pain and suffering to experimental animals"; (refinement).

The application of all 3Rs is presently implanted in the drafting procedure of regulatory direction both at the European and at International Conference on Harmonization. Pertaining to non-clinical testing necessities for human medicinal products, over the past years, new in vitro procedures have been accepted for regulatory use via multiple and flexible approaches, either as pivotal, helpful, or exploratory mechanistic studies, wherever relevant. At the same time as the replacement of animal studies remains the decisive goal, the application of all 3Rs needs to be the focus. As such, approaches aiming at reducing or refining animal studies are and have been regularly implemented in regulatory guidelines, where applicable.

There are two main barriers to implementation of the 3Rs: one is regulatory and the other is scientific. The main regulatory hurdles are

- the lack of harmonization of regulatory requirements, worldwide
- the prudence of health authorities to accept deviations from established guidelines
- the complexity of regulatory changes that discourage and slow the development and implementation of alternatives to animal testing; this is one of the main reasons, that industries have not been able to fully implement alternative tests described in European pharmacopoeia

The key scientific hurdles are

- the inherent inconsistency of in vivo tests
- the fact that the in vivo tests are not validated as per ICH requirements
- the fact that the product quality attributes will likely be assessed differently when changing from an in vivo to an in vitro method

Consequently, a one-to-one comparison is often challenging and not essentially justified.

6.7   INITIATIVE TOWARD WORLDWIDE HARMONIZATION OF 3RS IN BIOLOGICALS

6.7.1   PERSPECTIVES OF THE WHO ON ATT AND POTENCY TESTS

Based on a review of the WHO's perspectives on safety tests and potency testing reviewed in 2012, the WHO supports replacing, reducing, and refining animal testing for the development, production, testing, and characterizing of vaccines for human consumption [27]. A lot release of any final lot of vaccines developed before 1999 was conditioned on an innocuity test, including the first requirement for pertussis vaccination [28] and the first requirement for tetanus and diphtheria vaccines [29]. There has, however, been some flexibility within WHO guidelines regarding how the test should be performed since 2000. It is recommended, e.g., that the test for Haemophilus influenzae type B conjugate vaccines be omitted for routine lot release when good manufacturing practices are in place and consistency in production has been well established to the satisfaction of the national regulatory authority [30]. The recommendation for typhoid conjugate vaccines [31] as well as the recommendation for inactivated poliomyelitis vaccines [32] has been modified as "The NRA should agree to test the final lots of the vaccine for unexpected toxicity (also called abnormal toxicity). Whenever the NRA is satisfied that consistent production and reliable good manufacturing practices have been established, this test can be omitted from routine lot release."

6.7.2   EUROPEAN PARTNERSHIP FOR ALTERNATIVE APPROACHES TO ANIMAL TESTING (EPAA)

In association with the European Partnership for Alternative Approaches to Animal Testing (EPAA), the European Alliance for Alternative Approaches to Animal Testing organized a workshop on the theme: Modern science for better quality control of medicinal products: Toward global harmonization of 3Rs in biologicals. Members of the workshop decided that abnormal toxicity testing and animal batch safety testing should be enthusiastically encouraged to be removed from all appropriate legal necessities and guidance documents (WHO recommendations, country specific strategies, pharmacopoeia monographs) regarding biologicals' safety testing. Global convergence on scientific principles of the use of suitably authenticated in vitro tests for replacing in vivo techniques has been known as an overarching goal in order to aid global regulatory approval of non-animal methods for analyzing the potency of vaccines, such as tetanus, erysipelas, and diphtheria, vaccines for humans and pigs. An additional way of unifying regulatory approaches was through the establishment of scientific requirements for new assays. A key regulator and manufacturer should be included in the discussions early on. In order to facilitate international collaboration, manufacturers and responsible experts, e.g., at the European Directorate for the Quality of Medicines and Health Care of the Council of Europe or the European Medicines Agency, were invited to submit ideas.

6.7.3 IMPLEMENTING THE PRINCIPLE OF THE 3RS THROUGH THE INDIAN PHARMACOPOEIA

To promote the humane care of animals used in testing with the objective of providing specifications that enhance animal well-being, the Committee for the Purpose of Control and Supervision of Experiments on Animals (CPCSEA) was formed in 1964 under the Indian parliament's "Prevention of Cruelty to Animals Act, 1960" and then revived in 1998 [33].

It is recommended in many monographs to use the BET as a substitute to rabbit pyrogen testing; a few monographs also recommend in vivo pyrogen testing; and efforts are being made to apply the 3Rs strategy for the same (Table 6.2).

As part of the plan to keep pace with the current requirements, a validated in vitro test, such as BET, will be introduced as a substitute for the pyrogen test, where warranted and authorized. There are several monographs that describe in vivo potency testing methods, and these methods are being considered for replacement with in vitro methods using instrumentation or cell culture systems as part of the 3Rs strategy. If possible, these animal methods can be refined to reduce animal use or to produce a more humane outcome. As a result of its critical review of all

TABLE 6.2
List of Products Substituted or Alternative to the Pyrogen Test in the Indian Pharmacopoeia

Vaccines	Recombinant Products
• Typhoid polysaccharide vaccine Yellow fever vaccine (live)	• Insulin lispro
• Inactivated influenza vaccine (split virion)	• Insulin aspart
	• Insulin lispro injection
	• Isophane insulin injection
• Hepatitis A (inactivated) and hepatitis B (rDNA) vaccine (adsorbed)	• Erythropoietin-concentrated solution
	• Interferon alfa 2-concentrated solution
• Inactivated hepatitis A vaccine (adsorbed)	• Erythropoietin injection
• Inactivated influenza vaccine (whole virion)	• Erythropoietin for injection
	• Filgrastim injection
• Inactivated influenza vaccine (surface antigen)	• Filgrastim-concentrated solution
	• Human insulin
• Japanese encephalitis vaccine (human)	• Insulin aspart injection
• Poliomyelitis vaccine (inactivated)	• Biphasic insulin aspart injection
• Tetanus vaccine (adsorbed)	• Biphasic insulin lispro injection
	• Interferon alfa 2 injection
	• Interferon alfa 2b injection
	• Interferon beta 1a-concentrated solution
	• Recombinant streptokinase bulk solution
	• Recombinant streptokinase for injection

animal tests prescribed in the monographs, the IP encourages studies that lead to improvements in animal welfare. Facilitating the implementation of the 3Rs requires a collaborative approach between the IPC, regulators, manufacturers, and analysts.

6.8 CONCLUSION

The regulatory agencies require to conduct specific tests on biologicals to ensure their safety, purity, efficacy, and identity. To perform these safety and quality tests on the biologicals a large number of animals are used. In recent decades, national and international pharmacopeia have taken initiatives to safeguard animals, which is consistent with Russell and Burch's principle of the 3Rs: replace, reduce, refine. To get the most out of this principle, there is a need to substitute the existing with the technique that is more accurate, more reliable, should have less interassay variability, and can be completed in a shorter period of time. Furthermore, a new perspective will prerequisite to be rooted and established in order to address ingrained animal-based paradigms that dominate the sector. An effort of this magnitude, which is needed today more than ever, can only be achieved through the open collaboration of every stakeholder and involving as many regions and countries as possible in the progression of innovation, to ensure that the most advanced and newly developed methods no longer remain the exclusive domain of only a few regions or countries. An end result of such cooperation would be a more harmonized, one that aligns regulations between countries and regions, eliminates obsolete animal tests from pharmacopeia and regulations, and accepts alternative methods as quality control instruments.

CASE STUDY   PYROGEN TEST OF IMMUNOGLOBULIN IN RABBIT FOR QUALITY CONTROL

INTRODUCTION

Because patient safety is of the utmost significance in the pharmaceutical sector, the XYZ firm is committed to providing outstanding parenteral goods, such as immunoglobulin. These products are administered intravenously. Pyrogen tests are an essential component of quality control because they provide conclusive evidence that the product in question is free of any components that could cause a fever to develop. However, if fake immunoglobulin is used during the test, it may provide results that cannot be relied upon and may put patients in danger.

OBJECTIVE

The principal goals of this case study are to conduct an inquiry into the probable presence of spurious immunoglobulin during the pyrogen test done in rabbits for the purpose of immunoglobulin quality control and to put adequate processes into place. Additionally, the case study aims to put appropriate procedures into place.

METHODS

Test: the immunoglobulin product that is the focus of this investigation has been sterilized so that it can provide accurate findings in the pyrogen test. This was done in accordance with the standards set. The pyrogen test is performed on healthy adult rabbits that have been carefully selected in order to eliminate the potential of any underlying immunological problems. This is done so that the results of the test can be relied upon.

Baseline Measurement: it is necessary to take readings of each rabbit's baseline temperature in order to determine the temperature range that is considered typical for the body of each rabbit.

- Beginning at least 90 minutes before the injection, take a temperature reading every 30 minutes. This should continue until the injection is administered.
- Determine each rabbit's "initial temperature" by taking the average of the two temperatures that were obtained at intervals of 30 minutes beginning 40 minutes before the injection and continuing until the injection was administered.

Every single rabbit receives an intravenous injection of the material being tested (immunoglobulin), which is administered directly into its system. Following the administration of an injection, the individuals' temperatures are carefully observed and recorded at predetermined intervals throughout the subsequent 30 minutes.

In order to collect data, the temperature readings of each rabbit, as well as clinical observations and any signs that the rabbit was having a bad reaction. These notes will be retained during the entirety of the experiment.

RESULTS

The temperature of the three rabbits unexpectedly increased to more than 1.4 °C while they were being observed, while the temperature of rabbits unexpectedly increased to more than 0.6 °C. The experiment was repeated with five additional rabbits, and this time, a number of the rabbits suffered sudden temperature spikes of more than 0.6 °C. This was an unexpected result. The conclusion that can be drawn from this is that the experiment was not conducted correctly. Some of the rabbits have had sudden jumps in their body temperatures, which is a sign that the immunoglobulin product contains false immunoglobulin.

The significance of the quality control method was brought to light when it was discovered that a spurious immunoglobulin had been present during the pyrogen test. This finding brought to light the significance of the animal-based quality control testing.

CONCLUSION

During the pyrogen test of immunoglobulin in rabbits that was performed for the purpose of quality control, it was determined, after tedious research and the execution of preventative measures, that there was in fact counterfeit immunoglobulin present. The accuracy of the pyrogen test is ensured by the laboratory's strict adherence to rigorous standards, and improved sample validation processes maintain the immunoglobulin's purity and ensure that it is safe for patients to use. These two advantages are a direct result of carrying out the pyrogen test on the product in question.

REFERENCES

1. World Health Organization. WHO Expert Committee on Biological Standardization Fortieth Report [Internet]. Geneva: WHO: 1990. Annex-2, Requirements for diphtheria, tetanus, pertussis and combined vaccines (revised 1989), [cited 2022 Oct 10]. 87 p. Report no.: 800. Available from https://apps.who.int/iris/bitstream/handle/10665/39526/WHO_TRS_800_(part1).pdf;jsessionid=B55FCA6D1125F CDF5939967FD9E01152?sequence=1

2. Beken S, Kasper P, van der Laan JW. Regulatory acceptance of alternative methods in the development and approval of pharmaceuticals. Advances in Experimental Medicine and Biology 2016;856:33–64. doi: 10.1007/978-3-319-33826-2_3. PMID: 27671719.

3. De Mattia F, Chapsal JM, Descamps J, Halder M, Jarrett N, Kross I, Mortiaux F, Ponsar C, Redhead K, McKelvie J, Hendriksen C. The consistency approach for quality control of vaccines - a strategy to improve quality control and implement 3Rs. Biologicals. 2011;39(1):59–65. doi: 10.1016/j.biologicals.2010.12.001. PMID: 21277791.

4. European Pharmacopoeia. Edition 8.0. Vol. 1. Strasbourg: Council of Europe; 2013. Chapter-2.6.9. Abnormal toxicity; p.184. Available from https://archive.org/details/EuropeanPharmacopoeia80/page/n4/mode/1up.

5. Garbe JHO, Ausborn S, Beggs C, Bopst M, Joos A, Kitashova AA, Kovbasenco O, Schiller CD, Schwinger M, Semenova N, Smirnova L, Stodart F, Visalli T, Vromans L. Historical data analyses and scientific knowledge suggest complete removal of the abnormal toxicity test as a quality control test. Journal of Pharmaceutical Sciences. 2014;103(11):3349–55. doi: 10.1002/jps.24125. PMID: 25209378; PMCID: PMC4278562.

6. Hort EC, Penfold WJ. Microorganisms and their relation to fever: preliminary communication. Journal of Hygiene (London). 1912;12(3):361–90. doi: 10.1017/s0022172400005052. PMID: 20474498; PMCID: PMC2167401.

7. Daneshian M, Wendel A, Hartung T, von Aulock S. High sensitivity pyrogen testing in water and dialysis solutions. Journal of Immunological Methods. 2008;336(1):64–70. doi: 10.1016/j.jim.2008.03.013. PMID: 18474369.

8. Montag-Lessing T, Störmer M, Schurig U, Brachert J, Bubenzer M, Sicker U, Beshir R, Spreitzer I, Löschner B, Bache C, Becker B, Schneider CK. Probleme der mikrobiellen Sicherheit bei neuartigen Therapien. Die Quadratur des Kreises [Problems in microbial safety of advanced therapy medicinal products. Squaring the circle]. Bundesgesundheitsblatt Gesundheitsforschung Gesundheitsschutz. 2010;53(1):45–51. German. doi: 10.1007/s00103-009-0993-3. PMID: 20012926.

9. Seibert FB, The cause of many febrile reactions following intravenous injections. American Journal of Physiology. 1925;71(5):621–651. doi.org/10.1152/ajplegacy.1925.71.3.621

10. Martin WJ, Marcus S. Studies on bacterial pyrogenicity. 3. Specificity of the United States pharmacopeia rabbit pyrogen test. Applied Microbiology. 1964;12(6):483–6. doi: 10.1128/am.12.6.483-486.1964. PMID: 14239579; PMCID: PMC1058164.

11. Hoffmann S, Luderitz-Puchel U, Montag T, Hartung T. Optimisation of pyrogen testing in parenterals according to different pharmacopoeias by probabilistic modelling. Journal of Endotoxin Research 2005;11(1):25–31. doi: 10.1179/096805105225006678. PMID: 15826375.

12. Williams KL. Endotoxins: Pyrogens, LAL Testing, and Depyrogenation [Internet]. 2nd ed. New York: Marcel Dekker; 2001. 400 p. Available from https://archive.org/details/endotoxinspyroge111will

13. International Conference for Harmonization [Internet]. September 1999; London: Specifications: Test Procedures and Acceptance Criteria for Biotechnological/Biological Products. 17 p. Available from www.ema.europa.eu/en/documents/scientific-guideline/ich-q-6-b-test-procedures-acceptance-criteria-biotechnological/biological-products-step-5_en.pdf.

14. Doke S, Dhawale S. Alternatives to animal testing: a review. Saudi Pharmaceutical Journal. 2015;23(3):223–9.doi:10.1016/j.jsps.2013.11.002.

15. Greisman SE, Hornick RB. Comparative pyrogenic reactivity of rabbit and man to bacterial endotoxin. Proceedings of the Society for Experimental Biology and Medicine. 1969;131(4):1154–8. doi: 10.3181/00379727-131-34059. PMID: 4897836.

16. Park CY, Jung SH, Bak JP, Lee SS, Rhee DK. Comparison of the rabbit pyrogen test and Limulus amoebocyte lysate (LAL) assay for endotoxin in hepatitis B vaccines and the effect of aluminum hydroxide. Biologicals. 2005;33(3):145–51. doi: 10.1016/j.biologicals.2005.04.002. PMID: 16055344.

17. Ranganatha N, Kuppast IJ. A review on alternatives to animal testing methods in drug development. International Journal of Pharmacy and Pharmaceutical Sciences. 2012;4(5):28–32.

18. Hartung T. Human(e) Pyrogen Test Study Group. Comparison and validation of novel pyrogen tests based on the human fever reaction. Alternatives to Laboratory Animals. 2002;30(Suppl. 2):49–51. doi: 10.1177/026119290203002S07. PMID: 12513651.

19. Nakagawa Y, Maeda H, Murai T. Evaluation of the in vitro pyrogen test system based on proinflammatory cytokine release from human monocytes: comparison with a human whole blood culture test system and with the rabbit pyrogen test.

Clinical and Vaccine Immunology. 2002;9(3):588–97. doi: 10.1128/cdli.9.3.588-597.2002. PMID: 11986265; PMCID: PMC119983.

20. Rockel C, Hartung T. Systematic review of membrane components of gram-positive bacteria responsible as pyrogens for inducing human monocyte/macrophage cytokine release. Frontiers in Pharmacology. 2012;3:56. doi: 10.3389/fphar.2012.00056. PMID: 22529809; PMCID: PMC3328207.

21. European Pharmacopoeia. Edition 8.0. Vol. 1. Strasbourg: European Directorate for the Quality of Medicines & Healthcare (EDQM); 2013. Chapter-2.6.30. MONOCYTE-ACTIVATION TEST; p.217. Available from https://archive.org/deta ils/EuropeanPharmacopoeia80/page/n4/mode/1up.

22. Meigs L, Smirnova L, Rovida C, Leist M, Hartung T. Animal testing and its alternatives - the most important omics is economics. ALTEX. 2018;35(3):275–305. doi: 10.14573/altex.1807041. PMID: 30008008.

23. Hendriksen C, Arciniega JL, Bruckner L, Chevalier M, Coppens E, Descamps J, Duchêne M, Dusek DM, Halder M, Kreeftenberg H, Maes A, Redhead K, Ravetkar SD, Spieser JM, Swam H. The consistency approach for the quality control of vaccines. Biologicals. 2008;36(1):73–7. doi: 10.1016/j.biologicals.2007.05.002. PMID: 17892948.

24. Schutte K, Szczepanska A, Halder M, Cussler K, Sauer UG, Stirling C, Uhlrich S, Wilk-Zasadna I, John D, Bopst M, Garbe J, Glansbeek HL, Levis R, Serreyn PJ, Smith D, Stickings P. Modern science for better quality control of medicinal products "Towards global harmonization of 3Rs in biologicals": the report of an EPAA workshop. Biologicals. 2017;48:55–65. doi: 10.1016/j.biologicals.2017.05.006.. PMID: 28596049.

25. European Pharmacopoeia. Edition 8.0. Vol. 1. Strasbourg: European Directorate for the Quality of Medicines & Healthcare (EDQM); 2013. Chapter-2.6.33. RESIDUAL PERTUSSIS TOXIN; p.217. Available from https://archive.org/deta ils/EuropeanPharmacopoeia80/page/n4/mode/1up.

26. Viviani L, Halder M, Gruber M, Bruckner L, Cussler K, Sanyal G, Srinivas G, Goel S, Kaashoek M, Litthauer D, Lopes da Silva AL, Sakanyan E, Aprea P, Jin H, Vandeputte J, Seidle T, Yakunin D. Global harmonization of vaccine testing requirements: making elimination of the ATT and TABST a concrete global achievement. Biologicals. 2020;63:101–105. doi: 10.1016/j.biologicals.2019.10.007. PMID: 31699501.

27. Shin J, Lei D, Conrad C, Knezevic I, Wood D. International regulatory requirements for vaccine safety and potency testing: a WHO perspective. Procedia in Vaccinology. 2011;5:164–170. doi:10.1016/j.provac.2011.10.015

28. World Health Organization. WHO Expert Committee on Biological Standardization sixteenth report. [Internet]. Geneva: WHO: 1963. Annex-1, Requirements for pertussis vaccine (requirements for biologicals substances No. 8), [25 p. Report no.: 274. Available from http://apps.who.int/iris/bitstream/handle/10665/40582/WHO_TRS_274.pdf;jsessionid=C809AD9B616C2E7032EA3D10BC21C70E?sequence=1 1963: Annex 1

29. World Health Organization. WHO Expert Committee on Biological Standardization seventeenth report. [Internet]. Geneva: WHO: 1964. Annex-1, Requirements for diphtheria toxoid and tetanus toxoid (requirements for biologicals substance No 10). 25 p. Report no.: 293. Available from http://apps.who.int/iris/bitstream/handle/10665/40609/WHO_TRS_293.pdf?sequence=1

30. World Health Organization. WHO Expert Committee on Biological Standardization Fourty-Ninth Report. [Internet]. Geneva: WHO: 2000. Annex-1, Recommendations production and control of Haemophilus influenzae type b conjugate vaccines. 27 p. Report no.: 897. Available from www.who.int/publications/i/item/94120897X

31. World Health Organization. WHO Expert Committee on Biological Standardization sixty-fourth report. [Internet]. Geneva: WHO: 2013. Annex-3, Guidelines on the quality, safety and efficacy of typhoid conjugate vaccines. 101 p. Report no.: 987. Available from https://apps.who.int/iris/bitstream/handle/10665/129494/TRS_987_eng.pdf?sequence=1&isAllowed=y

32. World Health Organization. WHO Expert Committee on Biological Standardization Sixty-Fifth report. [Internet]. Geneva: WHO: 2015. Annex-3, Recommendations to assure the quality, safety and efficacy of poliomyelitis vaccines (inactivated). 89 p. Report no.: 993. Available from https://apps.who.int/iris/handle/10665/173739

33. Ministry of Agriculture and Formers Welfare, Governments of India. The Committee for Control and Supervision of Experiments on Animals (CCSEA) [Internet]. Available from https://cpcsea.nic.in/Content/57_1_Introduction.aspx

7 Good Manufacturing Practices in Quality Control

Bhartendu[1], Priyanshi Singh[2],
Supriya Shukla,[2] and Gauri Misra[2]
[1]Syngene International Limited, Bangalore, India
[2]National Institute of Biologicals, Ministry of Health
and Family Welfare, Government of India, Noida –
201309, India

7.1 BACKGROUND OF GMP

Until the 1960s, the basic methods and formulae were relied on the individual's experience and were considered as the operating procedure, which became inadequate with the increasing batch sizes [1]. Later in 1971, The Medicine Inspector of the Department of Health and Social Security of England, compiled a guide to Good Manufacturing Practices (GMPs) that is also regarded as the Orange Book [2, 3]. While in 1963, the GMP regulations were implemented to be obeyed in all manufacturing facilities in the United States. In 1978, USFDA established the GMP regulations and issued the United State CFR Chapter 21, which was enforceable by law unlike the advisory guide issued by the UK [4, 3]. The second addition of the "Orange Guide" was published in 1977 and later in 1983, the third edition was launched. The new edition of the Orange Guide was published by the Medicines and Healthcare products Regulatory Agency (MHRA) [4].

As a result of GMP systems in recent times, the incidence of safety problems is less frequent [4], but in the past there were a series of incidents that brought up the concept of GMPs. In 1902, The Biological Control Act was implemented to check the safety and purity of vaccines and other biological products, after the horse serum used to formulate the antitoxin for diphtheria was contaminated with live tetanus, leading to the death of children because of tetanus. In 1906, the Food and Drug act was launched to make the selling of contaminated food and meat illegal. Later in 1935, a company called Massengill included a poisonous component (diethyl glycol) in the oral solution of sulfanilamide, that caused the death of around 107 people including children, which led to The Food, Drug and Cosmetic Act that demanded companies to prove their product safe before selling in market. Again in 1941, around 300 people died after taking sulfathiazole tablets contaminated

DOI: 10.1201/9781032697444-7

with phenobarbital, which happened due to manufacturing deficiencies in the plant. This incident forced the FDA to revise the regulations and restriction for manufacturing and quality check, and these control standards were later called Good Manufacturing Practices (GMPs), officially in 1962 an amendment to the US Food, Drug and Cosmetic Act [4, 3].

7.1.1 OVERVIEW OF WORLDWIDE GMP

Good Manufacturing Practices (GMPs) are followed by over 100 countries in the world after it was implemented in the 1960s by the World Health Organization (WHO). Along with the GMPs issued by the WHO, several countries have designed guidelines that are relevant to their local needs enclosing the analogous subject matter and design [5]. Amongst them, several national and international regulatory guidelines have been officially known across the globe, be in the form of regulations, guides, codes, or the directives, for pharmaceutical manufacturing [6]. Some of the major examples that are commonly referenced and are quite persuasive are "The US Current Good Manufacturing Practices for Finished Pharmaceuticals regulations (The US cGMP)" and "The Guide to Good Manufacturing Practice for Medicinal Products of the European Union (The EC GMP Guide)." Other regulations as per regional requirements comprises of "Pharmaceutical Inspection Convention (PIC)—guide to GMP for pharmaceutical products", "European Economic Community (EEC)—guide to GMP for medicinal products," and "Association of South-East Asia Nations (ASEAN) GMP - general guidelines" and many more that replicates the US GMPs [7]. There are some regulations that are stated by the manufacturers of Indian Pharmaceuticals regarded as "Schedule M – Good Manufacturing Practices and Requirements of Premises, Plant and Equipment for Pharmaceutical Products" under The Drugs and Cosmetics Act and Rules, 2005 [7, 8]. These regulations have been augmented by several illustrative pieces of information on exclusive topics over the past many years. The factors responsible for the revisions of the guidelines includes the emerging manufacturing strategies, variations in the product requirement, and traceability methods and advancement of the facilities that has obligated the nations to upgrade their Acceptance Level of Protection (ALOP) on demand of the legislators and retailers to put rigorous quality checks for the suppliers [7].

7.2 GOOD MANUFACTURING PRACTICES (GMPs) AND OTHER FDA GUIDELINES

Good Manufacturing Practices (GMPs) refer to "the component of quality assurance that determines the products are produced in a reliable manner with a controlled quality paradigm to make them suitable as per the marketing authority obligation for their proposed use across the globe" as per stated by the World Health Organization (WHO) [8, 9]. In general, GMPs are a set of rules and procedures that aim for a safe and hygienic product manufacturing that includes all the production activities like validation of critical manufacturing steps, approving written procedures and guidelines, modification of technologies and equipment, availability of appropriate premises for storage and packaging, trainings for production and quality control personnel and maintaining proper documentation for traceability of the products [8, 9]. The GMP ensures that each time the product is made, it follows the same protocol and same specifications that are prescribed and approved as Standard Operating Protocols (SOPs), illustrating the steps to be performed in the entire production and quality control check [9]. The insight to follow Good Manufacturing Practices (GMPs) developed with the realization that the "final product quality testing" is not enough to assure the product or a drug quality. Rather, it must be guaranteed at each step involved in the manufacturing [10]. In alliance with several national regulatory bodies of different countries and the Pharmaceutical Industry, the GMP guidelines have been implemented by several international organizations and institutions for the assurance of efficacy, safety, and quality that are obligatory for marketing authorization (MA) [2].

7.2.1 Fundamentals of Good Manufacturing Practices (GMP) Regulation

In common language, regulation is known as a law. All federal laws in the United States have been codified or organized in a way that makes it simpler to locate a specific statute. The Code of Federal Regulations (CFRs) is a compilation of all federal laws that have been published in the Federal Register by executive departments and agencies of the federal government. There are 50 titles in this code, each of which represents a major area of government regulation. Chapters are further separated into each title. The chapters are then divided into sections that focus on regulatory fields. The Federal Register is where amendments and additions are initially published. The newest version of any regulation shall be determined likewise codified law and the Federal Register [12].

The regulations defining Good Manufacturing Practices for finished pharmaceutical products are included in Parts 210 and 211 of CFR Title 21. To promote their goods in the United States, all manufacturers are required to abide by these rules. A preapproval inspection of the manufacturing facility is one of the final steps in approving an application when a company submits one to market a product in the United States through a New Drug Application (NDA), Biological License Application (BLA), or other product application. Assuring compliance with the GMP rules is one of the main goals of this examination. Every application approval includes preapproval inspections. As a result, a company should anticipate ten inspections if there are ten applications outstanding. It is still necessary to conduct another inspection even when the production facility has already undergone inspection.

Any manufacturing facility that creates a product or items sold in the United States is also subject to inspection by the Food and Drug Administration (FDA).

These inspections happen without warning. When an inspector visits a plant, the manufacturer is required to allow them access without delay [13].

GMP, or Good Manufacturing Practices, is a system of regulations and norms that ensure the quality, safety, and consistency of pharmaceutical, biotechnology, and medical device goods. Regulatory authorities such as the FDA in the United States and the European Medicines Agency (EMA) in the European Union enforce GMP rules [14].

7.2.2 ROLE OF QUALITY MANAGEMENT UNIT

A department inside a company that is responsible for maintaining the quality of goods and services is called a Quality Management Unit (QMU). The main purpose of a QMU is to establish quality standards, observe performance, and identify areas for development and execute corrective action when necessary. Generally, a QMU works closely with other departments inside the company to develop quality control procedures and implement quality management systems [17].

Some major roles of a QMU are explaining the organizations quality goals and objectives and ensuring that these objectives are communicated and understood across the organization. This unit is also responsible for monitoring quality performance, such as produced goods' quality, customer satisfaction, and process variations. A QMU recognizes the areas for improvement and takes corrective action when necessary [14]. External and internal audits or inspection is also conducted by this unit to ensure the quality standards and regulations. Audits are helpful in identifying any refusal and allows for corrective actions to be taken. QMU works towards improvement within the organization [18] and provides required education and training to employees on quality management principles, process, and techniques, this action helps to ensure that all staff members understand their role in maintaining and improving quality standards.

Apart from all that, the main goal of QMU is to ensure that the organization consistently delivers exceptional products or services that meet or exceed customer demands [12].

7.2.3 SELF-ASSESSMENT AND INTERNAL AUDITS

ISO (International Organization for Standardization) provides guidelines for audits in quality control through its standard ISO 19011:2018, titled "Guidelines for auditing management systems." While ISO 19011 does not specifically focus on quality control audits, it provides general guidelines for auditing management systems, including those related to quality control.

To ascertain if quality-related actions and results adhere to established standards, laws, or requirements, audits in quality control are methodical, impartial examinations that are done. The main goal of audits is to make sure that products and processes adhere to relevant standards and guidelines and satisfy the specified quality levels. There are different types of audits in GMPs, including internal audits, self-assessment, and external audits. Audits in quality controls are performed against established criteria, which can include industry standards, regulatory requirements, company policies, and best practices. These criteria serve as benchmarks to evaluate the effectiveness of quality control activities.

Before conducting an audit, a detailed plan is developed, outlining the scope, objectives, audit criteria, and audit methods. The plan ensures that the audit is focused, comprehensive, and aligned with the organization's quality goals. The audit process typically involves several steps, including conducting an opening meeting, collecting and reviewing relevant documentation, performing on-site inspections, interviewing personnel, and assessing compliance with the audit criteria.

In the context of GMPs, self-assessment and internal audits are important activities to ensure compliance with regulatory requirements and maintain product quality and safety. Self-assessment involves an internal evaluation of a company's compliance with GMP regulations and its own quality system. The purpose of self-assessment is to proactively identify any gaps or areas of improvement in processes, procedures, and systems. It helps an organization to ensure that its operations align with established standards and to mitigate any risks that could impact product quality. During self-assessment, various aspects of the manufacturing facility and quality systems are reviewed, including documentation, facility and equipment, personnel and process controls.

Self-assessments are typically conducted by internal quality assurance or compliance teams. The findings from the self-assessment are used to identify areas of improvement, initiative corrective actions and enhance overall compliance and quality system of the organization.

External Audits

External audits play a crucial role in quality control providing an objective assessment of an organization's processes, systems, and products/services. These audits are conducted by independent third-party entities, often certified auditors typically trained professionals with expertise in auditing methodologies and the relevant industry standards or auditing firms who are not directly involved in the operations being assessed. Its aim is to evaluate an organization's compliance with established quality standards, regulations, and industry best practices. They verify that the company's quality control processes are effective, consistent, and aligned with the desired outcomes.

External audits are performed against specific standards and regulations that apply to the industry's operations. These standards may be international standards such as ISO 9001 (Quality Management System), ISO 14001 (Environmental Management System) or industry specific regulations and guidelines. External audits typically follow a structured process that includes planning, on-site assessment, reporting, and follow-up. The audit plan outlines the objectives, scope, and methodology. During the on-site assessment, auditors review documents, interview personnel, and conduct inspections to gather evidence. The audit finding and recommendations are documented in an audit report, which may highlight non-conformities, areas for improvement, and commendable practices. Audits provide several benefits for quality control; they help organizations identify gaps and weaknesses in their processes, leading to improved efficiency, product/service quality, and customer satisfaction. Audits also enhance credibility and trust in the organization's operations, which can be advantageous for attracting customers, business partners, and investors. In some cases, successful completion of an external audit may lead to certification or accreditation. Certificate is formal recognition that an organization's quality management system complies with specific standards. It demonstrates the organization's commitment to quality and can provide a competitive advantage in the marketplace. It is important to note that the specific details of external audits may vary depending on the industry, country, and applicable standards [15].

7.3 ELEMENTS OF GMP IN INDUSTRIES FOR QUALITY CONTROL

7.3.1 GENERAL

Good Manufacturing Practice (GMP) is the verified guideline sets that are applicable for various fields of business activity, which are designed to guarantee the explicit results. For each business type, the directive guidelines are elaborated in their relevant codes and guidebooks established through experience [8]. The various elements that encompass GMP are explained below.

Organizational and Infrastructural

Good Manufacturing Practices ensure the presence of proper management and the adequate infrastructure of any enterprise. The management of the organization plays a key role in providing all the necessary and apt resources, such as human resources, business development, project management, materials, and supply chain management, financial, equipment, and their maintenance, quality control units and many more to instigate and uphold the quality management and expand its efficacy [16, 11]. The organization is deemed to be the best operative when the management is effective and coordinated. Human resources are responsible for the recruitment of the staff while the allocations of the tasks are the sole responsibility of project management. While other management groups ensure the delivery of all the necessary resources, materials, and instruments [16]. The quality management team ensure the accomplishment of all product quality goals that requires the commitment by the staff at all stages in the organization and through the suppliers and distributors as well [10]. Furthermore, a quality control unit is the most important part of the organization that has the authority to accept or reject any component, drug product container, labeling or packaging material, and/or any measures or arrangements that can affect the quality, purity, or strength of the product [2]. Functional area management keeps a track of personnel training before engaging them in manufacturing, processing, or holding of the products.

The individuals must get educated, trained, and experienced in their functional areas in considerations to cGMP regulations under the qualified supervisors before performing any task.

GMP regulations also ensure the infrastructural setup of the organization includes the premises and the equipment and facilities present within. They must meet the expectations and comply with all the rules in accordance with the procedures to be performed at the site to abate the risk of errors and contaminations. There are two major areas of concern while designing a facility unit that is external environment, which must be acquiescent to the location such that it must not acquire any infestation or contamination of any type or likely water damages. Such facilities can be alleged incompatible to produce any kind of drug or food product. Prior to the relevant construction of the facility unit, certain factors need to be well thought-out such as ample space expansion, accessibility to water, fuel, waste-stream removal, transportation accessibility for personnel and materials, and the vicinity for other unfavorable activities that can cause potential contamination. The design and the layout of the facility is another important concern referred to as the internal environment that must curtail the chances of mix-up and contaminations and allows effective housework, maintenance, and proper operations. While constructing a facility for a manufacturing plant, the choice of material is decided as per the characteristics of the manufacturing process. For example, the wall positions should not hamper the material and personnel movement and must be made of high-quality concrete blocks or gypsum board with a plaster-like finishing. The choice of floor must endure the chemical contact and be durable for a long span, while the ceilings must be made of non-brittle, non-combustible, and non-friable lay-in acoustical panels with proper light fittings, sprinkler heads, and air-vents to avoid dust accumulation. The facilities must also possess adequate heating, ventilation, and air-conditioning (HVAC) for proper temperature and humidity controls [2].

The equipment and instruments must also comply with the rules to diminish the risk of errors. Their surfaces must have even and polished design with no rough weld or joints to harbor any contamination and must allow the detailed cleaning of the equipment since the traces from previous product batch is deplorable [3]. The maintenance and cleaning of these equipment must comply with the written standard procedures [2].

Current GMP in Production and Process

Good Manufacturing Practices in the production operations define the clear objectives and procedures in accordance to obtain a product with obligatory quality in accordance to the marketing authorizations (MA) [17]. For each product, an inclusive master manufacturing instruction (MMI) is provided, which is based on the trails carried out to institute the formulation and procedure for the factory production and is verified for their product yields in a consistent manner with final product specifications. These instructions can also be modified later based on the extended trails or any significant changes in the raw material while ensuring that the MMI is still being followed and is still significantly representing the specified final product [5]. Before starting the production procedures, it is mandatory that all the concerned personnel are aware of what to do, when to do, and how to do. Also, there must be a check to validate that the processing unit is contamination free, all the materials available are accurate, the instruments are sterilized and are ready to use, and the setup procedure is appropriate [18,5]. During the production processes, all the facilities must have an instructions guide that is readable for the operators [18].

There are two major subsections that represents the current Good Manufacturing Practices (cGMP) for production that includes the written standard protocols approved by the responsible person that needs to be followed in the entire process as explained above and the documentation of the procedure that is performed during the process [16]. The maintenance of the records for all the production procedure including any deviations from the actual instructions is mandatory and should be accurate and justifiable [18]. These records ensure that the manufacturing is done under the controlled physical factors like pH, temperature, humidity, flow rate, and pressure in a cautious manner and the product is non-contaminated and is proficient at avoiding any unwanted microbial growth. In addition to these conditions, there are several other written production procedures that ensure that the batch has been formulated with the commitment to provide a hundred percent of the established active ingredients and the components for the product manufacturing have been measured accurately. The final products are thus released in the market only after they get the approval from the responsible personnel, until then they are segregated and stored in the appropriate conditions, which are followed until their packaging and delivery [16].

7.3.2 Prohibition of Contaminations in Production

The occurrence of any kind of contamination, may it be because of improper sterilization of the equipment or due to mix-ups of the components, it leads to the production of undesired and non-specified final products that cannot be used further. The major threat of cross-contamination originates from the unrestrained release of sprays or dust particles, from residual contaminations left on the equipment, intruding insects or other factors like operator's clothes or body parts. Hence, during any production process it is made sure that all the equipment and apparatus have been sterilized as per the standard operating protocols and made sure that there is no source of contamination [2]. The proper air control is examined to provide the supply of suitable quality air and the dissemination of the dust particles is taken care of, especially while dealing with the dry components and raw material. The other alternative to avoid the cross-contamination is to carry out the production of a specific product in a dedicated and self-contained facility, or by conducting the production at specified time intervals after cleaning the facility by set procedures. Also, only the authorized personnel must be allowed to enter the facility after wearing the protective clothing to avoid the entrance of any contaminant in the facility. As per the GMP guidelines, the production areas designated to produce the susceptible products must undergo regular environmental monitoring and should be cleaned and sterilized [17].

7.3.3   PACKAGING, LABELING, AND DISTRIBUTION

The packaging and labeling of the product are as vital as its manufacturing, including the selection of raw material. The primary packaging material is referred to as the material that comes into direct contact with the product (e.g., ampoule, vials, stoppers, packet, etc.), while the printed labeled material protecting the product as well as the primary container is referred to as the secondary packaging material. The selection, purchase, and release of these packaging materials should be done with a great level of attention and with proper approvals for their anticipated usage [3]. The primary packaging materials (glass, plastic, foil, textiles, metal, etc.) must be tested for its compatibility with the product with a record that it does not allow any alterations in the product [19]. The packaging of the product ensures its preservation and enhances the storage life by controlling the local environment conditions that can deteriorate the product quality. It also provides the containment that makes the storage and transportation of the product suitable. In general, packaging can be considered as ideal when it bestows zero toxicity, high product visibility, resists the leaching or product degradation with a low cost, easy availability, and strong marketing appeals [18].

To make the product packaging effective, it must provide clear, accurate, and necessary information addressing the legal and the commercial demands. This makes the labeling a vital part of product packaging that can be applied directly to the primary container or secondary packages. The labeling error is the major reason for product withdrawal from market, thus the labeling of a product must avoid any kind of falsification about the ingredients and the effects of the product, not even inadvertently [16, 19]. The information to be notified on the labels must stick to the regulatory requirements and must be cross-checked for its authenticity. Labels must contain the necessary details, including the name, lot number, date of manufacturing and expiry, and all the ingredients present in the product along with its use and other general instruction, if applicable. The labeling material of each specific product must also be stored separately to avoid any mix-ups and the leftover labels from any batch must also be discarded to avoid their accidental misusage [19, 20]. Once packaging and labeling is done, the product must be stored in an arrangement that provides the "batch segregation" and follows FEFO, "first expiry, first out" ensuring the wet cleaning of the floors without harming the packed materials [3]. Also, the storage rooms for the final packed products until their distribution must have controlled temperature, humidity and light to maintain the product quality and strength [16].

Once all quarantined final products get the approval for its distribution, the product which is oldest approved goes out first. The proper records are maintained for each lot by the quality control before their approval and release that permits only those products in the market that have qualified the standard requirements as per the regulatory authorities of that region [16]. The records for the product distribution also govern the recall of the product from market, if needed [19].

7.4   QUALITY SYSTEM AND RISK MANAGEMENT APPROACHES

Risk is sometimes characterized as debatable future events, both good and bad, that could have an impact on the accomplishment of a company's aim. An efficient risk management and internal control system is one of the factors that can assist a firm reach its goals and objectives. Setting an organization's strategy, a unit's goal, or managing day-to-day operations are just a few examples of where risk management can be applied. There are various types of risk like strategic risk, hazard risk, financial risk, and operational risk. The discussion of risk management techniques that follows will canter mostly on how they might be used in pharmaceutical manufacturing processes.

Methods for managing risk have been utilized for a while in a variety of fields, such as investments, finance, safety, and pharmaceuticals. The FDA started using quality risk management in August 2002, albeit it is still a relatively new idea in the pharmaceutical business.

The fundamental tenet is that the assessment of the risk to quality is based on the patient risk. Anything that has a high impact or is very close to the product will be high risk from a manufacturing perspective. One high-risk activity that requires compliance is the weighing of active components in pharmaceutical production processes. There are at least three different categories of risk to consider in the field of GMP compliance. Naturally, the risks associated with patients and products must always be considered. Another sort of risk to consider is collective risk. It is possible to identify a number of hazards or failures that, while they may not all seem substantial or have an immediate impact on the product, may do so when taken together. Figure 7.1 is a representation of risk management process (from ICH Q9).

The project's first stage is risk assessment, which includes risk identification, analysis, and evaluation. It is essential to begin the procedure with a precise problem description or risk inquiry. This will make it easier to collect data and information and select the appropriate tools for analysis. Three questions are commonly used to identify risks: what could possibly go wrong? The probability that something will go wrong is what. And what is the gravity or repercussion? Focusing on the last two inquiries and calculating the risk and detectability that go along with them constitute risk analysis. A qualitative (high to low) or qualitative (numerical probability) technique can be used to evaluate risk. The established criteria are compared to the danger that has been discovered and examined. The outcomes of the risk assessment phase are a risk estimate for a quantitative approach or a risk range for a qualitative approach.

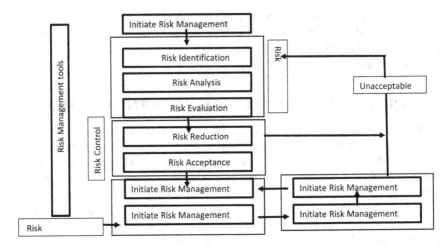

FIGURE 7.1   Risk management process.

The aim of the second phase, known as risk control, is to lessen or eliminate the risk to a level that is acceptable. Risk management focuses on four issues: does the risk exceed what is reasonable?

What can be done to lessen, manage, or even eliminate the risk? What is the ideal ratio of resources, benefits, and risk? Are there any additional hazards because of these efforts? Risk control includes risk reduction (measures taken to lessen or eliminate the risk) and the choice to accept that risk. In some circumstances, it might not be possible to eliminate the risk, but prompt corrective measures could bring it down to a manageable level or ensure its detection.

The third phase is risk communication. There ought to have been communication between decision-makers and stakeholders if a team has been working on the issue. For other parties involved in or impacted by the choices and modifications, nevertheless, a more formal process of notice may be required.

The last phase is the risk review. Particularly when a formal approach is used, the outcome of the risk management process should be documented. Reviewing the findings and output is necessary to identify fresh information and lessons. Monitoring the adjustments and outcomes will allow you to determine whether you need to restart the risk management process to deal with anticipated or unforeseen situations. A continuous quality management process should include risk management [21].

7.5   QUALIFICATIONS AND VALIDATION

Each pharmaceutical business should determine, in accordance with GMP, what qualification and validation work are necessary to demonstrate that the crucial elements of their operation are under control. A validation master plan should clearly identify and include the essential components of a company's certification and validation procedure. Qualification is the process of demonstrating and documenting that a specific system, instrument, equipment, or facility is suitable for its intended purpose and meets predefined requirements. It involves a series of tests, checks, and evaluations to verify that the system or equipment operates correctly, consistently, and within predefined parameters. The main purpose of qualification is to establish confidence that the system or equipment will perform as expected throughout its intended lifecycle. Validation is the process of establishing documented evidence that a system, process, or method consistently produces results or outcomes that meet predetermined acceptance criteria. Validation is particularly crucial for processes involved in the production of goods or services, especially in regulated industries like pharmaceuticals, medical devices, food, and aerospace.

Any facet of operation, including substantial alterations to the location, amenities, tools, or procedures, that could have an impact on the product's quality either directly or indirectly, needs to be qualified and verified. Validation and qualification should not be viewed as one-time activities. Following its initial deployment, they should establish a continuing program that is built around an annual review. The company's essential paperwork, such as the quality manual or validation master plan, should make clear its commitment to upholding continuing validation status. Validation should be performed under clearly specified authority. Validation studies must be carried out in accordance with established and authorized protocols because they are a crucial component of GMP. A written report detailing the findings noted and judgments made should be created and kept. The outcomes of the completed validation should serve as the foundation for the creation of processes and procedures. The validation of analytical test methods, automation systems, and cleaning practices needs to receive special consideration [22].

7.5.1 Validation of Laboratory Equipment's

The applicability and functionality of the data collection tools have a big influence on how accurate chemical and physical measurements are. Creating a pragmatically designed validation program for lab equipment of various complexity levels is difficult for any laboratory. However, the putting of such a program into action is very beneficial because it guarantees that instruments are suitable for their intended purpose and meet performance standards. These guarantees are necessary for compliance with Good Manufacturing Practices (GMPs) and good laboratory procedures (GLPs).

Validation of lab equipment refers to the process of verifying and documenting that the equipment used in laboratory setting consistently produces accurate and reliable results. It is an essential part of ensuring the quality and integrity of scientific experiments and analyses [22]. The validation process typically involves several steps like assurances that the instrument is appropriate for its intended use are the primary goal of laboratory instrument validation. Documented proof that the system consistently functions in accordance with established standards for the applications it is intended for supports the assurance [23]. Verify that the equipment is installed correctly and in compliance with the manufacture's specification, facility requirement, and safety guidelines. This includes checking the physical setup, connections, power supply, and any necessary calibration or adjustments and this complete process is known as installation qualification (IQ). Test and verify that the equipment operates as intended within its specified range. This involves conducting functional tests, assessing instrument control and parameters, and verifying that the equipment meets performance criteria and predefined acceptance criteria, this is called operational qualification (OQ) apart from IQ and OQ performance qualification (PQ) also done to validate that the equipment consistently performs as expected and generates accurate results under normal operating conditions. This typically involves conducting a series of tests, experiments, or comparisons against reference standards or known samples to demonstrate the equipment's accuracy, precision, sensitivity, linearity, and repeatability. Maintenance and calibration of lab equipment is also important to ensure that the equipment remains in optimal working condition. This includes routine inspection, cleaning, calibration checks, and any necessary adjustments or repairs [22]. Maintain comprehensive documentation throughout the validation process, including protocols, test results, calibration certificates, maintenance records, and any deviations

Validation is an ongoing process, and equipment may require periodic revalidation to ensure continued performance and compliance. Validation procedures may vary across industries, such as pharmaceuticals, medical devices, food manufacturing, and scientific research [24].

7.5.2 Analytical Methods: Validation and Quality Control

The assessment and technical reliability demonstrate compelling evidence that the monitoring system is adequate for the intended purpose in terms of priority study, reliability, and consistency of the test impact.

In different terms, the effects can be complicated whether the same method is applied in another laboratory over a long period of time in the world, under the same models and varying the assumptions [25].
Every technique needs to be validated:

- Before using on a regular basis
- When the parameters of analysis are altered, such as when the technique, the intended concentration range, or the sample matrix are modified
- Whenever an existing process is modified

Prior to preparing to validate the technique, it is crucial to gather pertinent information about analysis requirements.

- To be identified components
- Expected concentration levels
- Necessary level of detection and measurement
- Sample matrix nature
- The kind of analytical method to be applied
- Required level of accuracy and precision [24].

Analytical technique is a chain of movements and investigation to show that every technique which is used produces accurate findings. Some usually analytical techniques encompass comparing elements like accuracy, variety, specificity, agility, detection, and quantification limits and so on.

- **Quality Control Samples:** quality manipulation samples, including standards, controls and blanks, are used to evaluate the analytical method and instrument performance over the years. These samples are sorted by relevant concentration or analyte deficiencies and test samples conducted a study to verify the accuracy and precision of the technique.
- **Instrument Performance Verification:** regular validation of the overall performance of assessment tools is essential to maintain reliable results. This includes learning tests, including equipment suitability testing, calibration verification, detector sensitivity tests, and other equipment-specific checks to ensure that the instrument operates within the appropriate overall performance parameters [26].
- **Internal Quality Control:** in the context of interest management, statistical methods are used to control the research process. Control charts in the form of Lewy-Jennings charts are used to track the performance of key parameters over the years, including precision and accuracy. Deviations from mounted manage limits may indicate capacity problems in technique or equipment [27].
- **Proficiency Testing:** the proficiency test requires participation in external interlaboratory research applications, where labs recruit blind samples for research to compare with those obtained through lab participation, provide objective assessment of lab performance, and consider potential areas used to calculate the improvement accuracy: reference standards or calculated samples can be analyzed and compared with the method and results to assess accuracy [28].
- **Precision:** it assesses the reproducibility and reproducibility of the method. Repeatability measures the variability when a sample is analyzed twice in a short period of time, usually with the same analyzer, using the same instrument. Reproducibility measures the variability between analyzers or laboratories of the same type.
- **Specificity/Selectivity:** it assesses how accurately the method is able to measure the analysts of interest in the presence of potential interference.

This involves examining the response of attitudes to the various factors that may be present in the model matrix.

- **Linearity:** indicates whether the method yields conclusions that can be consistent with the researcher's focus in the chosen area. Linearity can be assessed with the aid of analyzing samples at different concentrations and plotting calibration curves.

- **Range:** define the lowest number that can be estimated by the method. This involves reading samples in different perspectives and ensuring consistent results, where desired [29].

- **Limit of Detection (LOD) and Limit of Quantification (LOQ):** the LOD is always the lowest analyte concentration that can be separated from the background noise of the analytical method, but concentrations may not always be determined with accuracy and precision. This is the apparent concentration if the signal is stronger than background noise LOD calculations are used. The LOD is then expressed as the multiple of the standard deviation of the blank signal (usually 3 or 2). Analytes with concentrations below the LOD are considered to be below the detection limit of the method because they have not been detected consistently. The analyte with the lowest concentration that can be quantified with some reliability and repeatability is known as the limit of quantification, or (LOQ). They can tell that someone is there. The LOQ is measured using calibration standards with known concentrations of analyte and is usually exceeded by the LOD. The LOQ is defined as the number (usually 10 or 3) of the standard deviation of the response of the calibration standards.

- **Robustness:** analyzes the robustness of the channel looking at small changes in parameters, such as pH, temperature, or mobile phase composition. This standardized approach involves introducing small changes and monitoring the impact on outcomes [28].

- **System Suitability:** ensure that the entire analytical system works, including instrument suitability, chromatographic resolution, peak symmetry, and detector response. Regular system requirement tests are performed to ensure that the method is a continuous operation.

- **Stability:** checks the stability of the analyte in the sample matrix and during sample storage and analysis. Stability studies involve the analysis of samples under storage conditions for a specified period.

- **Interference and Matrix Effects:** identifies possible interferences and matrix effects that may affect the accuracy and reliability of the method. It involves the analysis of samples known to contain interference or spiked matrices [30].

7.6 DOCUMENTATION

Documentation is a vital part of the Good Manufacturing Practices in any functional manufacturing facility that curbs a check on the quality assurance system of the facility and thus the product safety [8, 11]. The objective to implement the documentation practices is to consider all the undertakings in the plant to warrant good hygiene by establishing policies, monitoring the operations and activities, controlling the products and recording all the information during the process of product manufacturing to minimize the threat of errors ascending from oral interface. Documentation helps in keeping track of complete batch history including the raw material consumption and for the final product as well. This in turn, becomes a dynamic part for audits to map out the component history as well as the procedures followed to produce the final product [5]. It is thus essential to stress upon developing the appropriate procedures and instruction guidelines and relevant templates for accurate compilation of the records. The design of documentation is specific as per each business stage of the organization and are accessible in multiple forms, such as paper-based or electronic, which are governed by the quality assurance specialists for their reliability and coherence [8, 11]. Hence, the documentation for the GMP has been categorized as per their requirements such as for implementation of policies for the organization, for the specifications like instructions and procedures, for scheduling out the tasks to be accomplished at a particular interval, and especially for the recording of all the data generated during and after the manufacturing to have a track of all the activities performed [5]. The most common and needful documents include a Quality Manual that explains the regulations that a company is bound to follow, a Policy Booklet explaining the implementation of the GMP viewpoints, a Site Master File for manufacturing activities, Standard Operating Protocols (SOPs) instructing the operational procedures for all the activities carried out in organization and Logbooks for recording the usage and calibrations of the instruments and records of other critical activities, such as cleaning, solution preparations, etc. And above all, the Lab Notebooks (LNBs) that are used by the manufacturing departments to record each step of the activity including the batch number and date and time for each step done, which are reviewed and kept protected for any future cross-references [3].

The organization that fails to uphold the appropriate records and the documentations are put on hold for many of the profits of the GMP [5]. Thus, it is necessary to ensure that all the documents are designed, reviewed, and distributed among the organization with utmost care and are relevant to marketing authorities (MA). The documents once generated must be approved and dated by the responsible person, which are non-changeable without the consent of the reviewer. The documents must contain the explicit content that should be readable and must undergo regular review cycles to be kept updated. Any amendments made should be signed along with the reason, date, and time, and it must be ensured that the outdated documents are not being used furthermore. Regarding the data record, it should be entered in the record books as and when any step is performed during manufacturing for its significant traceability. In modern times, most of the data is stored electronically, which makes it easily accessible, thus it is important to also ensure that only designated people have the authority to enter and modify the data in order to avoid any conflicts, by restricting it with passwords and other restrictions

[17, 31]. Any sort of deviation from the above explained documentation ethics can debilitate the prominence of the quality assurance functions of the organization and thus might fail to sustain the market needs. That is why, documentation is always an emphasized crucial facet of Good Manufacturing Practices (GMPs) [31].

7.7 CONCLUSION

The execution of guidelines for Good Manufacturing Practices (GMPs) and their successive revision with modernization of the techniques has proved to be advantageous to provide the enhanced quality, safety, and efficacy of the manufactured product [11]. GMP aims to fabricate the quality of the product at each step of the operation that includes the organization, personnel training, providing proper facilities and equipment, controlling production, packaging and distribution processes and documentation as well [18]. Worldwide, many nations have laid the laws to instigate the GMP guidelines amongst the manufacturing companies, organizations, or other institutes, whether public or private. Each nation has even crafted their own GMP regulations that still aims to safeguard the quality of the product and thus safety of the purchaser [3]. At present, the product manufacturing skills are evolving with the enhanced technologies and thus it makes this important to keep the efforts ongoing to improvise the current status of the GMP by setting new goals and regulations heading to a better quality of life for society, by indorsing pubic and individual health [10, 11].

REFERENCES

1. Basnet P, editor. Promising pharmaceuticals. BoD–Books on Demand; 2012 May 23.
2. Gad SC, editor. Pharmaceutical Manufacturing Handbook: Production and Processes. Hoboken: John Wiley & Sons; 2008.
3. Chaudhari V, Yadav V, Verma P, Singh A. A review on good manufacturing practice (GMP) for medicinal products. PharmaTutor. 2014;2(9):8–19.
4. World Health Organization, WHO Expert Committee on Specifications for Pharmaceutical Preparations. Quality assurance of pharmaceuticals: Meeting a major public health challenge.
5. Blanchfield JR. Good manufacturing practice (GMP) in the food industry. In Handbook of Hygiene Control in the Food Industry 2005; pp. 324–47. Cambridge: Woodhead Publishing.
6. Covarrubias CE, Rivera TA, Soto CA, Deeks T, Kalergis AM. Current GMP standards for the production of vaccines and antibodies: an overview. Frontiers in Public Health. 2022;10:1021905.
7. Ojha A, Shukla R, Bhatt S, Singh R, Shukla TP. Quality assurance and quality control in formulation development. International Journal of Pharmaceutical Research and Applications. 2023;8(1):1168–74.
8. Sikora T. Good manufacturing practice (GMP) in the production of dietary supplements. In Dietary Supplements 2015;pp. 25–36. Poland: Woodhead Publishing.

9. Chaloner-Larsson G, Anderson R, Egan A, Da Fonseca Costa Filho MA, Gomez Herrera JF, Supply V, World Health Organization. A WHO guide to good manufacturing practice (GMP) requirements. World Health Organization; 1999.

10. Patel KT, Chotai NP. Pharmaceutical GMP: past, present, and future–a review. Die Pharmazie-An International Journal of Pharmaceutical Sciences. 2008;63(4):251–5.

11. Gouveia BG, Rijo P, Gonçalo TS, Reis CP. Good manufacturing practices for medicinal products for human use. Journal of Pharmacy & Bioallied Sciences. 2015;7(2):87.

12. Nally JD (editor). Good Manufacturing Practices for Pharmaceuticals. 6th ed. CRC Press; 2007.

13. Schlauderaff A, Boyer KC . An overview of food and drug administration medical device legislation and interplay with current medical practices. Cureus. 2019;11(5):e4627.

14. USP Quality Review No. 40 Revised 6/94. http://usp.org/patientSafety/newsletter/ quality/Review/qr401994-06-01c.html, accessed Aug 25, 2006.

15. Grant EL, Leavenworth RS. Statistical Quality Control. 7th ed. New York: McGraw-Hill.

16. Tetzlaff RF. Validation issues for new drug development part II, systematic assessment strategies. Pharmaceutical Technology 1992;16(10):84.

17. Vesper JL. Defining your GMP training program with a training procedure. BioPharm 2000;13(11):28–32

18. Guidance for Industry, Sterile Drug Products Produced by Aseptic Processing— Current Good Manufacturing Practice. U.S. Department of Health and Human Services, Food and Drug Administration; September 2004.

19. U.S. Department of Health and Human services, U.S. Food and Drug Administration, Pharmaceutical cGMPs for the 21st century — A risk - based approach, Final Report — Fall 2004, September 2004

20. International Organization for Standardization (ISO), (2002), Guidelines for quality and/or environmental management systems auditing, ISO 19011:2002, ISO, Geneva.

21. Nally JD, editor. Good Manufacturing Practices for Pharmaceuticals. Boca Raton: CRC Press; 2016.

22. World Health Organization. WHO guidelines on good manufacturing practices (GMP) for herbal medicines. World Health Organization; 2007.

23. Rahman MS, editor. Handbook of Food Preservation. New York: CRC Press; 2007.

24. Witcher MF. Introduction to Biomanufacturing. Encyclopedia of Industrial Biotechnology: Bioprocess, Bioseparation, and Cell Technology. 2009:1–8.

25. Gad SC, editor. Pharmaceutical Manufacturing Handbook: Regulations and Quality. Hoboken: John Wiley & Sons; 2008.

26. Nally J, Kieffer R, Stoker J. From audits to process assessment—the more effective approach. Pharmaceutical Technology, 1995; 19(9):128.

27. FDA compliance policy guide section 130.000, FDA access to results of quality assurance program audits and inspections (CPG 7151.02), available www.fda.gov/ ora/ compliance_ref/cpg/cpggenl/cpg130 - 300.html, accessed Dec. 5, 2006.

28. Ellison SLR, Barwick VJ. Using validation data for ISO measurement uncertainty estimation. Part 1. Principles of an approach using cause and effect analysis. Analyst 1998;123:1387–92.

29. Dehouck P et. al. Determination of uncertainty in analytical measurements from collaborative study results on the analysis of a phenoxymethylpenicillin sample. Analytica Chimica Acta 2003;481:261–72.

30. Rösslein M. Evaluation of uncertainty utilising the component by component approach, Accreditation and Quality Assurance 2000;5:88–94.
31. Armishaw P. Estimating measurement uncertainty in an afternoon. A case study in the practical application of measurement uncertainty Accreditation and Quality Assurance 2003;8:218–42
32. Segura M, Camara C, Madrid C, Rebollo C, Azcarate J, Kramer GN, Gawlik BM, Lamberty A, Quevauviller P. Certified reference materials (CRMs) for quality control of trace - element determinations in wastewaters. Trends in Analytical Chemistry (2004);23:194–202.
33. Analytical Methods Committee. Uncertainty of measurement: Implications of its use in analytical science. Analyst 1995;120:2303–8 .
34. Küppers S. Is the estimation of measurement uncertainty a viable alternative to validation? Accreditation and Quality Assurance 1998;3:412–5.
35. Association of Official Analytical Chemists (AOAC) International (2000), Method validation programs (OMA/PVM Department), including Appendix D: Guidelines for collaborative study procedures to validate characteristics of a method of analysis, available.
36. Patel KT, Chotai NP. Documentation and records: harmonized GMP requirements. Journal of Young Pharmacists. 2011;3(2):138–50.

TABLE 7.1
Major Countries and their GMP Regulation Authorities

Countries	Regulatory Authority	Product Types Inspected
United States	Code of Federal Regulations	Bulk Pharmaceutical Chemicals, Finished Pharmaceuticals
Europe		Finished Pharmaceuticals, Active Pharmaceutical Ingredients
Canada	Health Canada	Finished Pharmaceuticals, Active Pharmaceutical Ingredients
Brazil	National Agency for Sanitary Surveillance, ANVISA	Finished Pharmaceuticals
Australia	Therapeutic Goods Administrations, TGA	Finished Pharmaceuticals, Active Pharmaceutical Ingredients
United Kingdom	Medicine and Healthcare Products Regulatory Agency, MHRA	Finished Pharmaceuticals
Germany	Ministry of Health, Labour and Welfare	Finished Pharmaceuticals, Active Pharmaceutical Ingredients
India	The Central Drugs Standard Control Organisation (CDSCO)	Pharmaceutical and medical devices
South Africa	Medicines Control Council	Finished Pharmaceuticals

8 The Role of Analytical Methods in Quality Control of Biologicals and Stability Testing of Biological Products

Khushboo Choudhury[1] and Rashmi[1,2]
[1]National Institute of Biologicals, Ministry of Health and Family Welfare, Government of India, A-32, Sector-62, Noida – 201309, India
[2]Academy of Scientific & Innovative Research, Ghaziabad – 201002, India

8.1 BACKGROUND

The manufacturing process is essential for maintaining the product's accurate composition, efficacy, quality, and safety. Since it can be difficult to predict the consequences of changes in the quality attributes on the safety and effectiveness of the specified product, controlling the manufacturing process is essential for preserving the reproducibility of the manufacturing batches. The caliber of raw components used to make the drug compound (unformulated active ingredient) and drug product (formulated drug including additives) should meet quality standards suitable for its intended use, according to the International Council for Harmonisation (ICH) Q6B guideline [1].

Most biologics are intricate, higher-order structures and are large in size, with a molecular weight range of 1–1000 kDa. The majority of biologics are produced from living organisms, such as humans, animals, or microorganisms, which are naturally unpredictable systems. Modern biotechnology techniques are used during the production processes, which typically entail cell culture, harvest, purification, modification techniques, and filling. The procedure is frequently specific to the medicinal chemical and can be complicated. Biochemical molecules are heat-sensitive and prone to microbial and enzymatic contamination. Degradation would be more likely under harsh manufacturing circumstances [2]. These elements have an impact on the biologic drug's production procedure and quality requirements.

DOI: 10.1201/9781032697444-8

The raw materials used in the formulations should be free of contaminants or impurities that could disturb the product's quality and safety due to the manufacturing process. The base and final product should be of pharmacopoeial standards. To guarantee that the manufacturing process is controlled and reproducible, ample understanding of process design and its capacity is needed. In-process satisfactoriness standards are established at key points in the production process [3]. Early in the development process, provisional boundaries are established and information is acquired for all production batches. The limitations or specifications are then improved upon and supported for the clinical and commercial batches using the information gained. Guidelines on process-related considerations, in-process acceptance criteria and specifications, and Q7on GMP are provided in ICH Q6B [4]. Additionally, the US Food and Drug Administration (FDA) offer guidelines on process validation, fundamental ideas, and best practices.

8.2 ANALYTICAL METHOD DEVELOPMENT

An analytical method is designed to create and evaluate specific characteristics of the drug or drug substance in comparison to the established standards for acceptance of the new product. Analytical methods' and instrumentation should be founded on the scope and purpose intended for that method. Some of the considerations that could be assessed during development of analytical methods are linearity, specificity, limits of quantitation (LOQ), accuracy, precision, limits of detection (LOD), and range. The robustness of methods should be assessed in the early phases of development and characterization because this quality can assist in the choice of technique to submit for approval. The initial creation of analytical processes is based on a mechanical grasp of the fundamental approach combined with prior experience [4] (Figure 8.1). Early experimental data can be utilized to direct subsequent development. If development data help validate the method, you should include them in the method validation section.

To grasp the effects of varying fluctuations in parameters of analytical processes, an organized approach has to be adopted for the analytical method robustness study. The initial risk assessment should be followed with multivariate experiments. The effects of factorial parameters on method performance can be comprehended using such methods. Analyses of samples taken at different phases of the manufacturing

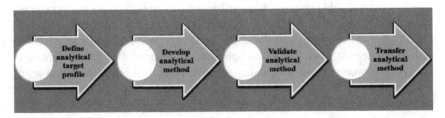

FIGURE 8.1 Workflow of analytical method validation in the characterization of biologics.

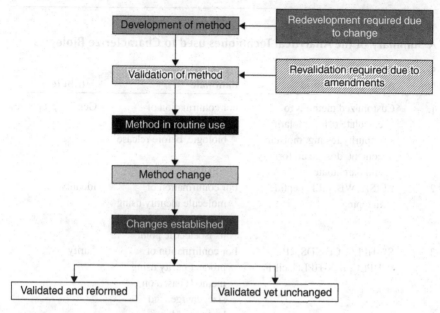

FIGURE 8.2 Development of an analytical method.

process, from the in-process stage through to the finished product, may be used to assess a method's performance. Evaluation of these techniques' performance can be done with the knowledge received from this research about the sources of method variance [5]. Figure 8.2 shows the flow of an established analytical method and its redevelopment in case of amendments to its SOP.

8.3 MONITORING OF ANALYTICAL METHODS

The guidelines for regulatory requirements for analytical testing of biologics are described in FDA, ICH as well as pharmacopeia, depending on the specificity of product type. For the characterization of biologic product, monitoring the manufacturing, batch consistency, and evaluating a range of analytical techniques for the measurement of purity, identity, strength, quality, potency, biological activity, and safety is required. Oftentimes, multiple analytical assays using cross-modal techniques, designed specifically for an analyte is required. Table 8.1 gives an overview of analytical methods that are currently used for characterization, stability testing, in-process, and final release of biologics.

8.4 CHARACTERIZATION METHODS FOR BIOLOGICS

Characterization methods for validation of biologics (Table 8.2) is usually classified into three broad categories:

TABLE 8.1

A Summary of the Analytical Techniques used to Characterize Biologics

Sr. No.	Analytical Method	Rationale	Attribute
1.	Customized methods to calculate pH, osmolarity, impurity testing, moisture content, dosage uniformity and particulates.	For confirmation of general properties of the biologic, before release	General properties
2.	ELISA, WB, ciEF, peptide mapping	For confirmation of molecule identity using specific antibodies, and its isoelectric point	Identity
3.	SE-HPLC, CE-SDS,RP-HPLC, IEX-HPLC, ciEF	For confirmation of product purity using methods based on size, charge, and hydrophobicity	Purity
4.	A_{280}, Bradford, BCA	For determination of protein concentration	Quantity
5.	Customized methods, residual host cell DNA PCR, CE-SDS, SDS-PAGE, residual HCP, Rp-HPLC, ciEF, IEX-HPLC, LC-MS/MS, light scattering, fractionation of impurities and characterization	For measurement of process and product-related impurities	Impurities
6.	Cell culture-based, receptor binding and cytotoxicity assays.	For measurement of biomolecular activity based on mechanism of action.	Potency/biological activity
7.	Microbiological contaminants, sterility testing, endotoxin, retrovirus, specific viruses, adventitious agents.	For ensuring the product is free and safe from viral and microbial contamination	Safety
8.	Binding assays, Western blot, ELISA, immunoreactivity assays	For ensuring optimal activity of antibody and antibody-based assays for determining avidity, affinity and immunoreactivity	Immunochemical properties

TABLE 8.2
Characterization Methods

Characterization Method	Type	Method and Principle
PCR (polymerase chain reaction)	Qualitative and quantitative	Quantitative PCR is a technique that involves labeling primers, oligonucleotide probes, or amplicons with molecules that fluoresce to track the buildup of amplicon as it is produced. Qualitative PCR is used to detect the presence or absence of a specific DNA product. It is a useful method to employ when PCR is carried out to detect a pathogen or for cloning purposes.
LC/MS-MS (liquid chromatography-mass spectrometry)	Quantitative	In mass spectrometry, the analyte molecules initially become charged (ionized), followed by ions and any fragment ions, created during the ionization process are subjected to analysis based on their mass to charge ratio (m/z).
NMR (nuclear magnetic resonance)	Qualitative and quantitative	This technique is used for direct observation of atoms through measurement of nuclear spin. It is used for the determination of concentration and purity of small molecules. In qualitative research, NMR is used for detection of unknown molecules.
CD (circular dichroism)	Quantitative	This technique is used to measure the absorption of circularly polarized light for investigation of structural rigidity of molecules. It is used to study biological structures and their interaction with other molecules.

(continued)

TABLE 8.2 (Continued)
Characterization Methods

Characterization Method	Type	Method and Principle
XRD (x-ray diffraction)	Quantitative	This technique measures the average position of atoms in a crystal, their chemical bonds, and disorder. These parameters can all be identified from the three-dimensional (3D) electron density image produced by diffracting x-rays from crystalline atoms in various directions. This is the most effective technique for figuring out the structures of macromolecular crystals, such as proteins, DNA, medicines, vitamins, etc.
FTIR (Fourier transform infrared)	Qualitative	This technique identifies various chemical bonds in molecules by creating an infrared spectrum that can analyzed for molecular fingerprinting.
Genetic stability testing	Qualitative	Used to demonstrate that the genetic sequence in an expression construct is stable throughout its lifecycle. This maintains the value and consistency of the new drug/cell product. This is maintained via ICH Q5B guidelines. For this purpose, next gen sequencing is the most reliable tool for this method.

8.4.1 Qualitative: for detection of the nucleic acid of interest
8.4.2 Quantitative: for detection of the levels of nucleic acid of interest
8.4.3 Limit testing: for detection of optimal levels of nucleic acid of interest

Some characterization methods for biologics are listed in the table below, including qualitative, quantitative, and semi-quantitative methods [6].

8.5 ANALYTICAL METHOD VALIDATION

8.5.1 PHARMACOPEIAL ANALYTICAL PROCEDURES

All types of analytical methods are validated to corroborate that the technique is the most suited for its intended use. Before embarking on validation studies, the objectives and methodology should be clearly demarcated and completely understood by the personnel performing them. All validation data has to be generated through standard operating protocols approved by the concerned authority followed by good manufacturing practices along with a detailed description of the methodology used and justified acceptance criteria, using capable instrumentation [7]. For drug substances, mixtures of analytes and/or product analytes in respective matrices need to be executed and developed.

8.5.2 VALIDATION CHARACTERISTICS

Even though not all test types can use all validation attributes, the majority of them can be classified under the following broad topics:

1. Specificity: the capacity to confirm the existence of the analyte in the presence of any components that would be predicted to be present.
2. Linearity: the capacity to generate test results that are (within a given range) directly proportional to the concentration (amount) of analyte in the sample.
3. Accuracy: the proportion of the known extra analyte in the sample that is detected by the test.
4. Range: a spectrum showing the range of an analyte's concentration in a sample.
5. Precision: a series of measurements are typically expressed as coefficient of variation, variance, or standard deviation.
6. Quantitation limit: the least amount of analyte that can be accurately and precisely determined quantitatively in a sample.
7. Detection limit: the lowest concentration of an analyte that can be detected in a sample.

Depending on where the product is in the development process, assays might be certified as GMP or non-GMP.

The principal source for suggestions and justifications of validation features for analytical processes is ICH Q2 (R1). A technique is considered to be a stability indicating test if it is a validated quantitative analytical approach with the potential to detect changes in the quality attribute(s) of the drug substance and drug product during storage. A range of trials should be carried out to show the specificity of a stability-indicating test. One of the challenges is dealing with real product samples that have either aged or have been stored in higher temperature and humidity settings after being stressed in the lab under various stress settings and injected with target analytes and all known interferences. To guarantee that criteria of accuracy and reliability are upheld, the testing of the analytical procedure must be done using data from properly listed submissions. Any minor modifications to the permitted conditions, including adjustments to the operating procedures, must be communicated to the regulatory authorities.

8.5.3 NON-PHARMACOPEIAL ANALYTICAL PROCEDURES

An analytical procedure's adequacy (using acknowledged standard references) should be confirmed under real-world usage circumstances. Information received in accordance with a verification process that demonstrates the suitability of analytical techniques for the drug product or drug substance should be included in submissions, in case of complaints raised. The verification protocol should ideally, but need not, include the following: (1) a detailed and exhaustive methodology that should be substantiated with fixed acceptance criteria; and (2) details pertaining to the methodology, such as the applicability of the reagent(s), apparatus, component(s), chromatographic settings, column, detector type(s), sensitivity of the detector signal response, system fitness, sample preparation, and stability.

Depending on the stage of the development program, analytical methods need to be created, qualified, and validated. According to FDA guidance on investigational new drug applications and ICH Q7 guidelines, analytical methods must be trustworthy, accurate, robust, and scientifically sound in order to be used for the intended purpose. Several guidance publications from the FDA and ICH may be used to identify analytical method requirements that are phase-appropriate. These include ICH Q7 and the FDA's current GMP for industry guidelines on phase 1 investigational pharmaceuticals [8].

Analytical information is acquired from early manufacturing batches and as the manufacturing process is being developed. On the basis of this data, suitable reference standards that are typical of the clinical batches are produced, along with initial acceptance standards for the intermediate and finished product. In the ICH Q6B and Q7 guidelines, primary and secondary reference standards and materials are specified and described. If accessible, the National Institute for Biological Standards and Control, the Centre for Biologics Evaluation and Research, the US Pharmacopoeia, the European Pharmacopoeia, the Indian Pharmacopeia, the Japanese Pharmacopoeia, the World Health Organization, or another source can provide reference standards. To identify the important qualities and be a representative of the clinical batches, reference standards that are created internally or from outside sources must be adequately characterized using orthogonal approaches.

8.6 LIFECYCLE MANAGEMENT AND POST APPROVAL CHANGES

In accordance with the idea of continuous improvement, analytical methods may evolve during the course of a product's lifecycle. Changes to analytical techniques may involve modifying or optimizing the current procedure or completely replacing the procedure with contemporary technology as additional process knowledge and analytical method data are obtained. Additionally, any adjustments to the product or production process will dictate a new evaluation of the analytical method's applicability. A bridging approach of partial or full validation and a comparative study of representative samples and standards may be needed if the current analytical method is changed or moved to a new location. Full validation of the new analytical technique is necessary if the analytical procedure's underlying concept has been totally altered.

8.7   STABILITY TESTING

This is a vital aspect towards overall control approach used to establish that biological products are of high quality, purity, safety, and potency. Compared to small molecules, biological and biotechnological products can degrade in more complex ways that may involve a variety of pathways, such as chemical decomposition (oxidation, deamination, etc.), fragmentation, aggregation, changes to high-order structure, and interactions with excipients, closure or container components, or other products [9]. In addition to the degradation of unstable products into lethal products, activity loss of up to 85% of that claimed on the label, as in the case of nitroglycerine tablets used for the treatment of angina and cardiac arrest, may lead to the death of the patient. Because of such concerns, it is now legally required to disclose information for certain stability tests to regulatory bodies prior to validation of new products [10].

8.7.1   STABILITY TESTING METHODS

The primary objective of stability testing is to give a reasonable level of confidence that the product will maintain an acceptable quality for consumption during its market presence and availability to patients, as well as until the patient consumes the last unit of the product [11]. These methods are divided into four types based on their objectives and procedural steps:

a.   Real-time stability testing
     The product is kept in precise storage settings and watched until it fails the specification. This knowledge is essential in determining the duration of time a product can be stored without significant deterioration [12].
b.   Accelerated stability testing
     The product's stability is assessed at higher temperatures (like 37°C), allowing the stability to be predicted or back-calculated at the normal storage temperature (like 4°C). During accelerated stability testing, stress variables such as moisture, pH, light, gravity, agitation, and packing are also used in addition to temperature [11].
c.   Retained sample stability testing
     The stability samples undergo testing at preset intervals; e.g., if a product has a 5-year shelf life, it is customary to test samples at various intervals such as 3, 6, 9, 12, 18, 24, 36, 48, and 60 months. The approach of collecting stability data from retained storage samples at fixed time intervals is referred to as the constant interval method [10].

d. Cyclic temperature stress testing

Utilizing product knowledge, this testing technique develops cyclic temperature stress tests to replicate actual market storage conditions. To stimulate the 24 hour rhythm on Earth, which the drugs on the market are likely to encounter during storage, the cycle period typically taken into consideration is 24 hours. For each specific product, it is advised to determine the maximum and minimum temperatures for the testing, considering factors like the product's recommended storage temperatures and particular physical and chemical degrading characteristics [10].

8.7.2 GUIDELINES FOR STABILITY TESTING

There are numerous regulatory guidance reports that need to be explored in order to develop a successful stability testing program. To ensure that accurate information is produced in favor of a new pharmacological product, these documents provide help on how to implement a stability program. These regulations were first published in the 1980s and were subsequently harmonized at the International Conference on Harmonization (ICH) to conquer market barriers and ensure product certification in other nations. In 1991, the European Commission, the United States, and Japan collaborated to form ICH, which also included contributions from the regulatory and commercial sectors. These rules are known as guidelines for quality, safety, efficacy, and multidisciplinary (QSEM). Because the ICH guidelines only covered novel drug substances, not the established ones that were previously available in the WHO umbrella countries, the World Health Organization (WHO) updated the guidelines in 1996. Furthermore, the harsh climatic conditions that can be observed in many nations were not covered by the ICH guidelines. In June 1997, the US FDA also released a guidance report titled "Expiration dating of solid oral dosage form containing Iron." Guidelines for global environmental stability research were also published by the WHO in 2004 [13]. Later, the ICH guidelines for veterinary goods were also extended. The India Drug Manufacturers Association has also released a technical monograph concerning stability testing of drug substances and products that are currently marketed in India [14, 15]. For active pharmaceutical ingredients (APIs), pharmaceutical products, formulations, and excipients, various test conditions and specifications have been developed in the guideline documents. As a result, stability study standards from the FDA, ICH, CPMP, and WHO must be followed, especially ICH Q1A (R2).

8.7.3 STABILITY TESTING PROTOCOL

Before initiating a stability test, it is essential to create a stability testing protocol, which serves as a written record outlining the key elements of a well-controlled and regulated stability test. The protocol depends on the type of drug substance, considering factors, such as inherent stability of the compounds, dosage form, and container closure system employed. The stability protocol should encompass essential details, including the number of batches, containers, and closures involving the storage conditions for containers, sampling time points, sampling strategy, test storage situation, test parameters, test procedure, and other relevant information [13].

To confirm the quality and efficacy of pharmaceutical products, stability testing is not only a legal necessity but also a crucial step. By determining the proper shelf life, storage conditions, and labeling instructions, it plays a crucial role in safeguarding patient health. As the healthcare sector continues to advance, stability testing will remain a crucial practice since it upholds the highest standards of product integrity and patient care.

8.9   ESSENTIALS OF EQUIPMENT VALIDATION – IQ, OQ, PQ

Before commencing process validation activities, it is necessary to complete the proper qualification of essential equipment and auxiliary systems. As per the FDA, "qualification refers to the set of activities carried out to establish that utilities and equipment are appropriate for their intended purpose and function properly. These activities are a prerequisite before manufacturing products on a commercial scale" [16]. Following this, as necessary, are various stages of qualification, including design qualification, factory acceptance test, a site acceptance test, installation qualification (IQ), operational qualification (OQ), and performance qualification (PQ). These depend on the function of the utility, equipment, or system [17]. Each IQ, OQ, and PQ procedure outlines the precise steps to take, the data to be recorded, a list of acceptable standards, and the materials, equipment, and documentation required to carry out the validation.

User requirement specifications (URS)
Manufacturers must create a document outlining the requirements for the item that has to be sourced. These requirements encompass specifications aimed at controlling potential GMP risks, fulfilling technical needs and referencing relevant documentation. When choosing the appropriate item from an authorized source and determining applicability during the consequent phases of qualification, the URS should be implemented [17].

Design qualification (DQ)
DQ process should furnish documented evidence demonstrating that the design requirements have been fulfilled and align with the URS.

Factory acceptance test (FAT) and site acceptance test (SAT)
Before moving on to the subsequent phases of qualification, it is essential to conduct the FAT and SAT when required to confirm the system's validity at the designated site. This has to be well documented [17].

8.9.1 Installation Qualification (IQ)

This documentation is essential for all the crucial processing equipment and systems used within the facility, such as the HVAC system, autoclave, or pH meter. The IQ of any equipment should encompass comprehensive details, including identification information, location, utility needs, and safety features. Every system or piece of equipment has an IQ protocol that includes information on its name, specifications, model and unique identification numbers, location, utility demands, connections, and necessary safety measures that should be documented. The IQ protocol should confirm that the purchased product meets the specified requirements and that relevant drawings, handbooks, spare part lists, vendor contact information, and addresses are available [18]. After the first IQ, requalification is required after any significant maintenance or whenever the equipment is upgraded. Regular quality assurance procedures should include requalification as well [19].

8.9.2 Operational Qualification (OQ)

Following the completion of each IQ protocol, an OQ is conducted. The goal of OQ is to assess if equipment performance is in compliance with URS within the manufacturer-specified operating ranges [19]. This entails evaluating all controls for normal operation, including alarm points, switches, displays, interacting controls, and any other operational indicators. The OQ document should include instructions for both static and dynamic tests to demonstrate the equipment's expected performance under typical conditions. It should also include a list of SOPs for operation, maintenance, and calibration, as well as information regarding operator training. For each operation, specifications and acceptability standards must be established. Information on equipment calibration, preoperational procedures, routine operations, and the corresponding acceptance criteria should all be included in the OQ document [18].

8.9.3 Performance Qualification (PQ)

Following the completion, assessment, and approval of both installation and operational qualifications, this phase of system and equipment validation is carried out. The PQ document outlines the method(s) for proving that a system or equipment can reliably operate and meet requirements during normal operation and, when necessary, under worst-case scenarios. The document should outline the necessary preliminary steps, the specific performance test(s) to be conducted, and define the test acceptance standards for each test. Additionally, supporting equipment utilized in the qualification process must undergo validation in order to comply with the PQ (e.g., the validation of the steam system must be completed before validating the autoclave) [18].

8.10   IQC CHARTS – NORMAL DISTRIBUTION, LEVEY JENNINGS CHART, WESTGARD RULES

Early detection of systematic and random errors is essential, and then every effort should be undertaken to reduce them. Specific statistical quality control (SQC) techniques are used in the approach for their detection, which can be broadly categorized into two groups.

Internal quality control (IQC): this includes all the SQC techniques used regularly by lab staff employing the materials and equipment in the lab. It primarily examines the method's accuracy (repeatability or reproducibility).

External quality control (EQC): this includes all the SQC techniques used periodically (i.e., monthly, bimonthly, twice a year) by lab staff with the participation of an external center like a referral laboratory, the diagnostic industry, etc. EQC primarily focuses on assessing the reliability of analytical methods in the lab. However, certain EQC schemes also evaluate both accuracy and precision aspects.

The metrics of IQC and EQC are derived from statistical science, such as the standard deviation index (SDI), coefficient of variation (CV), and Z-score. These metrics are graphically represented using statistical charts, commonly known as control charts [20].

8.10.1   Normal Distribution

The normal distribution, also referred to as the Gaussian distribution, is a widely utilized continuous probability distribution in probability theory. It holds great significance in statistics and finds extensive application in both the natural and social sciences. Its purpose is to show random variables that take on real values and whose underlying distribution is not known. Normal distributions are a crucial type of statistical distribution. The distribution chart is typically presented as a two-dimensional diagram with an x-axis and a y-axis. In this chart, the x-axis corresponds to the values of the observed variable, while the y-axis represents the frequency associated with each value (Figure 8.3). All normal distributions exhibit symmetry and possess bell-shaped density curves characterized by a single peak. The mean, which denotes the location of the density peak, and the

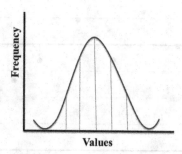

FIGURE 8.3   The normal distribution.

standard deviation, which denotes the extent or breadth of the bell curve, have to be addressed specifically when discussing any normal distribution [21].

8.10.2 Levey-Jennings Chart

In 1950, Levey and Jennings modified Walter Shewhart's original statistical control chart and brought it to medical laboratories as a statistical process control. Levey and Jennings suggested taking duplicate readings on the patient specimen as opposed to Shewhart's original suggestion, which involved taking a group of readings, computing the average and range, and subsequently graphing the mean and range on separate control charts. This was a challenging application because the measured constituent's true level fluctuated from specimen to specimen. A different method was created by Henry and Seaglove that involved repeatedly analyzing a stable reference sample and directly plotting individual values on a control chart. The control chart where individual values are directly plotted is widely recognized today as the Levey-Jennings chart. It serves the purpose of identifying both systematic and random analytical errors and estimating the magnitude of those errors. Typically, these charts are created with horizontal limit lines at various standard deviations, including 1, 2, 3, and occasionally 4 standard deviations (Figure 8.4). These charts can be created using z-values, which represent the mean and +/- 1, 2, or 3 standard deviations along the y-axis. Alternatively, they can also be created based on precise mean and standard deviation levels. The choice of representation depends on the specific requirements and preferences of the analysis. With Levey-Jennings charts, you have the ability to plot data in a sequential manner, run by run or level by level, and decide which data points indicate acceptable, "in-control" behavior and which points reflect unacceptable, "out-of-control" behavior [22]. By analyzing the plotted points on the chart, you can make informed judgments regarding the stability and quality of the process being monitored.

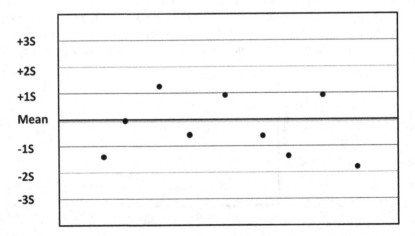

FIGURE 8.4   Levey-Jennings chart.

8.10.3 WESTGARD RULES

Westgard rules, devised by Dr. James Westgard, are a collection of statistical guidelines employed either independently or in conjunction to identify random and systematic errors (Table 8.3). These errors introduce measurement uncertainty, which is vital to acknowledge when comparing testing procedures or results

---

TABLE 8.3
Westgard Rules

1_{2SD} The rule serves as a cautionary measure (warning rule), prompting a thorough examination of the control data. To eliminate the possibility of a trend, it is important to consider control values from the previous run when a control measure exceeds the mean±2SD.

2_{2SD} The rule serves to identify systematic errors and is considered violated when two consecutive control values (both on the same side of the mean) surpass the same mean +2SD or mean -2SD limit.

4_{1SD} The rule serves to identify systematic errors and is considered violated when four consecutive readings surpass the same mean ±1SD. While the violation of this rule does not necessitate the rejection of the run, it should serve as a trigger for recalibration or equipment maintenance.

1_{3SD} This control rule is used to identify random errors, and its violation may indicate the presence of systematic errors as well. When a control value surpasses the mean ±3SD, it signifies that the assay run is out of control.

R_{4SD} This particular range rule is designed exclusively to identify random errors. It is applicable only within the current run. When one control measurement within a group surpasses the mean +2SD and another measurement exceeds the mean -2SD, the rule is considered violated.

10_X The rule serves to identify systematic errors and is considered violated when ten consecutive values consistently fall on the same side of the mean. The violation of this rule often signifies the degradation of assay reagents. It is typically applied across multiple runs and sometimes across different materials as well.

8_X The rule is considered violated when eight consecutive values consistently fall on the same side of the mean.

12_X The rule is considered violated when 12 consecutive values consistently fall on one side of the mean.

3_{1SD} The rule is considered violated when there are three consecutive control measurements that exceed the same mean ±1SD control limit and all of them fall on the same side of the mean.

6_X The rule is considered violated when six consecutive control measurements fall on the same side of the mean.

9_X The rule is considered violated when nine consecutive control measurements fall on the same side of the mean.

---

against each other or specified standards. These rules establish precise performance limits for a specific assay, ensuring the reliability of test outcomes [23]. They are symbolized by A_L. A denotes the number of control observations to be evaluated, while L represents the control limits [24].

8.11 RELIABILITY AND ROBUSTNESS

Robustness evaluation must be taken into account during the development process and depends on the technique being examined. This provides proof of an analysis' consistency with regard to additional alterations in the method's tested restrictions. If measurements are susceptible to changes in such settings, analytical circumstances should be carefully controlled, or a caution should be written into the protocol. To ensure that the analytical procedure's validity is sustained every time it is used, the robustness assessment should result in the formulation of a number of system suitability parameters (such as the resolution test).

8.12 CONCLUSION

Analytical method characterization is an essential key to quality control of biologicals. It is used to safeguard that analytical methods are fit for their projected purpose, and that they can provide accurate and reproducible results. Depending on the unique product type, regulatory requirements for analytical testing of biologics are provided by the ICH, global pharmacopeial, and FDA guidelines. These techniques are crucial for process and product pipelines in the early stages of development of biologics. The latest techniques in analytical method validation would help in improving the efficiency and effectiveness of the validation process. These techniques make it possible to validate analytical methods more quickly and easily, and to ensure that the validated methods meet the highest standards of quality.

REFERENCES

1. Rudge SR, Nims RW. ICH Q6B specifications: test procedures and acceptance criteria for biotechnological/biological products. ICH Quality Guidelines: An Implementation Guide. 2017:467–86.
2. Hellings P, Verhoeven E, Fokkens W. State-of-the-art overview on biological treatment for CRSwNP. Rhinology. 2021;59(2):151–63.
3. Golchin A, Farahany TZ. Biological products: cellular therapy and FDA approved products. Stem Cell Reviews and Reports. 2019;15(2):166–75.
4. Swartz ME, Krull IS. Analytical Method Development and Validation: CRC press; 2018.
5. Chauhan A, Harti Mittu B, Chauhan P. Analytical method development and validation: a concise review. Journal of Analytical & Bioanalytical Techniques. 2015;6(233):2.

6. Chirino AJ, Mire-Sluis A. Characterizing biological products and assessing comparability following manufacturing changes. Nature Biotechnology. 2004;22(11):1383–91.

7. Akhunzada ZS, Hubert M, Sahin E, Pratt J. Separation, characterization and discriminant analysis of subvisible particles in biologics formulations. Current Pharmaceutical Biotechnology. 2019;20(3):232–44.

8. Huynh-Ba K. Drug regulations and the pharmaceutical laboratories. Analytical Testing for the Pharmaceutical GMP Laboratory. 2022:1–25.

9. Ye J, Liu Z, Pollard D. ICH Q5B analysis of the expression construct in cell lines used for production of recombinant DNA-derived protein products. ICH Quality Guidelines: An Implementation Guide. 2017:337–44.

10. Bajaj S, Singla D, Sakhuja N. Stability testing of pharmaceutical products. Journal of Applied Pharmaceutical Science. 2012:129–38.

11. Kommanaboyina B, Rhodes C. Trends in stability testing, with emphasis on stability during distribution and storage. Drug Development and Industrial Pharmacy. 1999;25(7):857–68.

12. Pokharana M, Vaishnav R, Goyal A, Shrivastava A. Stability testing guidelines of pharmaceutical products. Journal of Drug Delivery and Therapeutics. 2018;8(2):169–75.

13. Zothanpuii F, Rajesh R, Selvakumar K. A review on stability testing guidelines of pharmaceutical products. Asian Journal of Pharmaceutical and Clinical Research. 2020;13(10):3–9.

14. Singh S. Stability Testing During Product Development in Jain NK Pharmaceutical Product Development. CBS Publisher and Distributors, India. 2000;10(3):272–93.

15. Huynh-Ba K, Zahn M. Understanding ICH Guidelines Applicable to Stability Testing. Handbook of Stability Testing in Pharmaceutical Development: Regulations, Methodologies, and Best Practices: Springer; 2009. p. 21–41.

16. Food and Drug Administration. Guidance for Industry Process Validation: General Principles and Practices, FDA, January 2011. 2011.

17. Voykelatos G. Good Manufacturing Practices (GMPs) and process validation in the pharmaceutical industry: an in depth analysis: Πανεπιστήμιο Πειραιώς; 2022.

18. Chaloner-Larsson G, Anderson R, Egan A, Da Fonseca Costa Filho MA, Gomez Herrera JF, World Health Organization. Vaccine S, et al. A WHO Guide to Good Manufacturing Practice (GMP) Requirements/Written by Gillian Chaloner-Larsson, Roger Anderson, Anik Egan; in collaboration with Manoel Antonio da Fonseca Costa Filho, Jorge F. Gomez Herrera. Geneva: World Health Organization; 1999.

19. Veselov V, Roytman H, Alquier L. Medical device regulations for process validation: review of FDA, GHTF, and GAMP requirements. Journal of Validation Technology. 2012;18(2):82.

20. Karkalousos P, Evangelopoulos A. Quality control in clinical laboratories. Quality control in clinical laboratories, applications and experiences of quality control INTECH Open Access Publisher. 2011:331–60.

21. Arzideh F. Estimation of medical reference limits by truncated Gaussian and truncated power normal distributions: Universität Bremen; 2008.

22. Westgard JO. Internal quality control: planning and implementation strategies. Annals of Clinical Biochemistry. 2003;40(6):593–611.

23. Dimech WJ, Vincini GA, Plebani M, Lippi G, Nichols JH, Sonntag O. Time to address quality control processes applied to antibody testing for infectious diseases. Clinical Chemistry and Laboratory Medicine (CCLM). 2023;61(2):205–12.

24. Fei Y, Wang W, Wang Z. A new internal quality control rules design tool in clinical laboratory-Westgard Sigma Rules. Journal of Modern Laboratory Medicine. 2015:149.

9 Regulatory Bodies
European Medicines Agency (EMA) and Pharmaceutical Inspection Co-Operation Scheme (PIC/S)

Satyajeet Singh, Manika P Sharma, and
Gauri Misra
National Institute of Biologicals, Ministry of Health and
Family Welfare, Government of India, A-32, Sector-62,
Noida – 201309, India

9.1 INTRODUCTION

The pharmaceutical industry is firmly directed to guarantee the security, adequacy, and quality of the medications. Regulators play an imperative part in observing and planning these controls. This chapter looks at two fundamental administrative bodies: the European Medicines Agency (EMA) and the Pharmaceutical Inspection Co-Operation Scheme (PIC/S).

The European Medicines Agency (EMA) is an organization of the European Union (EU) responsible for the logical survey, assessment, and administration of medications. The office works with national controllers and industry partners to guarantee medications meet the most elevated guidelines of safety, adequacy, and quality.

The EMA provides a centralized approval process for promoting authorization, oversees post-authorization safety monitoring, and supports research and development in healthcare. Its administrative specialist incorporates a noteworthy effect on the supply and use of medicines over EU member states.

The Pharmaceutical Inspection Co-operation Scheme (PIC/S) is a worldwide Good Manufacturing Practice (GMP) organization for the review of pharmaceutical facilities. PIC/S member nations mutually create and keep up benchmarks and methods for GMP inspections. These assessments guarantee that the pharmaceutical manufacturing process meets the most noteworthy measures, minimizing the risk of contamination, adulteration, or manufacturing failures.

DOI: 10.1201/9781032697444-9

PIC/S ensures the universal harmonization and coordination of GMP reviews by advancing the trade of information, skill, and best practices among administrative agencies. These points highlight the important role EMA and PIC/S play in pharmaceuticals. Their efforts help maintain health, provide safe and effective medicines, and support good manufacturing practices. The cooperation and collaboration supported by these regulatory bodies has a profound impact on the pharmaceutical industry, ensuring the safety and reliability of medicines worldwide. This section summarizes the important role played by the EMA and the PIC/S in the regulation of medicinal products. Their efforts help protect public health, provide safe and effective medicines, and promote Good Manufacturing Practices. The collaboration fostered by these regulatory bodies has had a significant impact on the pharmaceutical industry, ensuring the stability and safety of drugs worldwide.

Their efforts help to protect public health, provide safe and effective medicines, and promote Good Manufacturing Practices. The collaboration and cooperation fostered by these administrative bodies has had a significant effect on the pharmaceutical industry, guaranteeing the safety and soundness of drugs around the world.

9.2   EUROPEAN MEDICINES AGENCY (EMA)

9.2.1   Historical Overview

EMA was established in 1995 to harmonize drug regulation over the European Union (EU) [1]. This segment looks at the authentic advancement of the EMA, highlighting the key standards and administrative systems that led to its formation. The EMA is an organization of the EU responsible for evaluation and safety monitoring of drugs. It is headquartered in Amsterdam, Netherlands.

The EMA plays an important part in the appraisal and endorsement of drugs within the EU. Its primary goal is to protect public health by ensuring that medicines sold within the EU are secure, viable, and proficient. The organization works closely with national controllers in EU States and other partners such as pharmaceutical companies, specialists, and medical associations.

The EMA evaluates medicinal products based on data submitted by pharmaceutical companies. These assessments incorporate assessing the quality, safety, and viability of the medicines, and the risk-benefit balance. The organization's views and suggestions shape the premise for the authorization of medicinal products in the EU.

In expansion to its role, within the initial approval of drugs, the EMA screens the drug's safety, understanding, permitting the use of potent drugs. It routinely evaluates new information with respect to the safety of drugs and takes suitable actions, such as updating product information and even withdrawing approval of the drug. The EMA plays an important role in the administration of controlled drugs in EU states by ensuring that patients have access to safe and effective drugs. Its work has had a major impact on public health in Europe over the past.

9.2.2 Organizational Structure

The European Medicines Agency (EMA) is the European Union's (EU) regulatory agency responsible for the scientific evaluation, monitoring, and safety of medications. EMA's organizational structure is as follows [2]:

1. Management Committee/Board:
   - The Management Committee is EMA's most elevated decision-making body.
   - It comprises of representatives of all EU member states, the European Commission and other stakeholders.
   - The Management Board provides direction and oversight for the operation of the organization.
2. Executive Members:
   - Executive Members are appointed by the Management Board.
   - The Executive administrator is responsible for the day-to-day operation of the organization.
   - They ensure the implementation of Board decisions and policies.
3. Scientific Committee:
   EMA has several scientific committees of independent experts.
   - Committee for Medicinal Products for Human Use (CHMP): responsible for the scientific evaluation of medicinal products for human use.
   - Veterinary Medicines Committee (CVMP): evaluation of veterinary medicines.
   - Pharmacovigilance Risk Assessment Committee (PRAC): evaluates the risks and benefits of drugs.
   - Committee on Orphan Drugs (COMP): reviews of orphan drugs for rare diseases.
   - Committee on Paediatrics (PDCO): addresses issues with pediatric drugs.
   - Herbal Medicinal Products Committee (HMPC): provides guidance on herbal medicines.
4. Support Centers:
   - EMA has a range of support services to assist in the scientific evaluation and regulatory processes.
   - Human Drug Research and Development Support: provides scientific advice, orphan drug development and pediatric development support.
   - Veterinary Drug Research and Development Support Branch: provides support to veterinarians.
   - Scientific Advice and Orphan Drug Coordination Unit: coordinates scientific tips and orphan drug assignment.
   - Regulatory Affairs Unit: support systems and procedures.
   - Health Safety Department: monitors the safety and risk-benefit analysis of drugs.

5. Liaison Officers:
   - EMA has Liaison Officers from EU member states who act as liaisons between the organization and national authorities.
   - They facilitate communication and coordination between EMA and national authorities.

9.2.3 RESPONSIBILITIES AND FUNCTIONS

EMA is a regulatory body that plays a key part within the observing, direction, and evaluation of medications within the EU. The organization has a responsibility to ensure the efficacy, safety, and quality of the pharmaceuticals. The role and responsibility [3] of EMA are as follows:

Marketing Authorization

The EMA conducts the centralized approval process for EU drug registration. Evaluates quality, safety, and efficacy data from pharmaceutical companies. The organization considers all aspects of the drug, including drug design, clinical and non-clinical data, and the benefit-risk balance.

Based on these measures, the EMA makes a recommendation to the European Commission, which then grants or refuses final marketing authorization [4].

Pharmacovigilance

The EMA is concerned with the post-authorization safety monitoring of drugs. The agency works with government regulators, doctors, patients, and pharmaceutical companies to collect and review safety data. This includes evaluating adverse drug reactions and risks associated with drugs and implementing appropriate policies to protect public health. These actions may include updating product information, limiting restrictions, or even removing business authorization where the risks outweigh the benefits [5].

Advice and guidance: EMA provides scientific advice to pharmaceutical companies during drug development. This guidance helps companies optimize clinical trials, meet regulatory requirements and improve data quality. The organization also develops guidelines and recommendations for the pharmaceutical industry. These guidelines cover a wide range of topics, including the quality, safety, and efficacy of medicines, as well as pharmacovigilance and Good Manufacturing Practices.

Orphan Drugs

EMA supports the development and use of drugs for rare diseases through its Orphan Designation program. The agency grants an orphan drug designation for drugs used to treat, diagnose, or prevent rare diseases that affect a small number of patients. Orphan drug designation provides companies with incentives, including special marketing and regulatory approvals, to support the development of orphan drugs and to address the unmet medical needs of rare diseases.

Collaboration

EMA works with many stakeholders, including national regulators, patient associations, medical professionals and other international regulators. This collaboration aims to encourage the exchange of knowledge, to train experts and to facilitate the management of applications.

The organization coordinates with worldwide regulatory authorities and is committed to coordinating regulatory decisions with regulators outside the EU. Such participation and collaboration increase the efficiency and effectiveness of the regulatory process, facilitates access to medicine and contributes to patient safety.

9.2.4 REGULATORY PROCEDURES

The European Medicines Agency (EMA) manages the regulatory process [4, 6] for the approval and monitoring of medicines in the European Union (EU). The regulatory process [6] carried out by the EMA is as follows (Figure 9.1):

1. **Centralized process:**
   - The EMA harmonizes the centralized process [7] for the registration of drugs in the European Union.
   - The centralized procedure is mandatory for certain drugs, including biotechnology products, orphan drugs, and drugs for the treatment

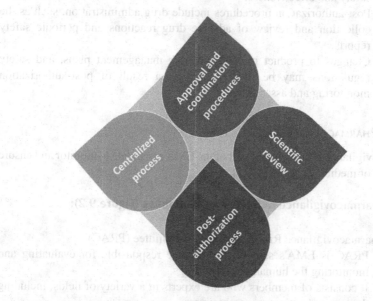

FIGURE 9.1 Regulatory procedures (EMA).

of human immunodeficiency virus (HIV), cancer, diabetes, and neurodegenerative diseases.

- As part of the central process, the European Commission grants a single marketing authorization that is valid in all EU countries.

2. Approval and Coordination Procedures:
   - Approval and proportionality procedures are applied for drugs that are not subject to centralized procedures.
   - In the recognition process, the medicinal product is first registered in an EU member state and then it can be extended to other member states by confirming the authorization according to the recognition law.
   - In the decentralized procedure, applications are sent to several member countries at the same time and national assessments are made by the respective countries in the same way.

3. Scientific review:
   - EMA's scientific team [6] plays an important role in the evaluation process.
   - The Committee for Medicinal Products for Human Use (CHMP) reviews the quality, safety, and efficacy of medicinal products for human use.
   - The Committee for Veterinary Medicinal Products (CVMP) evaluates veterinary medicinal products.
   - This group makes recommendations on the registration of drugs based on their scientific evaluation.

4. Post-authorization process:
   - Once the drug is approved, the EMA continues to monitor the drug's safety and effectiveness.
   - Post-authorization procedures include drug administration, such as the collection and review of adverse drug reactions and periodic safety reports.
   - Changes to product information, risk management plans, and safety regulations may be implemented as a result of post-authorization monitoring and assessment.

9.2.5 PHARMACOVIGILANCE

Pharmacovigilance is an essential part of the EMA's mandate to monitor and ensure the safety of medicines in the EU [5].

EMA's Pharmacovigilance Activities are as follows (Figure 9.2):

1. Pharmacovigilance Risk Assessment Committee (PRAC):
   - PRAC is EMA's scientific committee responsible for evaluating and monitoring the human safety of drugs.
   - It consists of members who are experts in a variety of fields, including doctors and patient representatives.

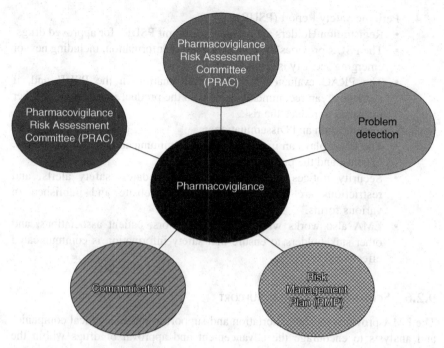

FIGURE 9.2   EMA's pharmacovigilance activities.

- PRAC evaluates data from a variety of sources, including voluntary reports, clinical trials, data and periodic safety reports submitted by pharmaceutical companies.
- It evaluates the risks and benefits of medications, advises on their use, and makes management recommendations to ensure patient safety.
2. Problem Detection:
   - The EMA uses a number of methods to identify indicators of drug-related safety concerns.
   - This process includes the identification of adverse drug reaction reports, large-scale database searches, data analysis, and the use of statistical methods.
   - PRAC conducts a comprehensive analysis of the signals found to determine if further investigation and management is needed.
3. Risk Management Plan (RMP):
   - As part of the licensing process, pharmaceutical companies must submit a RMP for certain drugs.
   - RMP outlines strategies and measures to identify, explain, and reduce the risks associated with drugs.
   - The EMA reviews and evaluates RMPs to ensure risk reduction measures are in place and the drug has a good benefit-risk ratio.

4. Periodic Safety Report (PSUR):
   • Registration Holders are required to submit PSURs for approved drugs.
   • The PSUR provides the EMA with safety information, including new or emerging security issues.
   • The PRAC evaluates the safety information in the PSUR and, if necessary, can recommend changes to the product information or other measures to reduce the risk.
5. Communication and Dissemination:
   • The EMA plays an important role in communicating safety to doctors, patients, and the public.
   • Security notices such as information updates, safety alerts, and restrictions are posted on the EMA website and published in various forms.
   • EMA also works with national regulators, patient associations, and other stakeholders to ensure that safety information is communicated effectively.

9.2.6 SCIENTIFIC ADVICE AND SUPPORT

The EMA provides logical exhortation and support to pharmaceutical companies and analysts to encourage the advancement and approval of drugs within the European Union (EU).

The EMA's advice and support is as follow:

1. Research Advice:
   • The EMA provides research advice to assist pharmaceutical companies and researchers at all stages of drug development.
   • Scientific advice may be sought before a marketing authorization is granted or during the development of a new medicinal product [8].
   • It can help participants understand regulatory requirements, design studies, and create documents required for marketing authorization.
2. Protocol Assistance:
   • Protocol assistance is a type of technical training provided by EMA to support the development of new drugs.
   • It focuses on early partnerships with pharmaceutical companies to develop drugs for rare diseases or unmet medical needs.
   • Protocol assistance for clinical trial development, including patient populations, endpoints, and study management can help to facilitate clinical trial improvement.
3. Pediatric Development:
   • The EMA provides guidance and support for the development of drugs in children.
   • The Committee on Pediatrics (PDCO) evaluates research on child development and makes recommendations on it [9].

- These recommendations will help ensure that the necessary research is done to establish evidence of the safety and efficacy of medicines for children.
4. Orphan Drug Designation:
   - The EMA provides Orphan Drug Designation for Drugs designed to treat rare diseases [10].
   - Orphan drug designation provides several incentives, including scientific and regulatory guidance, to encourage the development of drugs for rare diseases with limited treatment options.
5. Regulatory Support:
   - The EMA provides regulatory support to pharmaceutical companies and researchers to improve understanding of regulations and procedures.
   - This support includes guidance on many aspects of drug development and approval, including efficacy, non-clinical, and clinical aspects.

9.2.7 COLLABORATION WITH INTERNATIONAL PARTNERS

The EMA works with many international partners to advance international participation and improve regulatory standards for medicines [11, 12].
An outline of EMA's work with international partners:

1. Regulatory Cooperation with Non-EU Authorities:
   - EMA's work with non-EU authorities includes knowledge sharing, exchange of expertise, and coordination of management and processes.
   - The EMA collaborates with regulatory agencies in countries such as Canada (Health Canada), United States (U.S. Food and Drug Administration), Australia (Therapeutic Goods Administration), and Japan (Pharmaceuticals and Medical Devices Agency).
2. International Committee for the Harmonization (ICH) of Technical Requirements for Medicines for Human Use:
   - The EMA is a member of ICH, an international organization that creates and promotes harmonization after development, registration and approval by pharmacists [13].
   - EMA collaborates with the development and revision of the ICH process to align management practices with international standards.
3. European and International Collaboration on Medicines Evaluation:
   - The EMA collaborates with international partners through initiatives such as the International Coalition of Medicines Regulatory Authorities (ICMRA) [11, 14] and the Heads of Medicines Agencies (HMA).
   - These collaborations facilitate information sharing, joint management and coordination to increase efficiency and effectiveness in the monitoring and management of international medicine.

4. International Harmonization of Pharmacopoeia Standards:
   - The EMA collaborates with international Pharmacopeia organizations [15] such as the United States Pharmacopeia (USP) and the British Pharmacopoeia (BP) to harmonize pharmacopoeia standards.
   - This coordination helps to ensure that drug standards are consistent across regions.

9.2.8 Key Regulations and Guidelines

The EMA is responsible for setting up rules and regulations for the improvement, assessment, and management of medications in the EU. The main regulations and directives issued by the EMA are as follows:

1. Regulation (EC) No 726/2004:
   - This regulation establishes the legal framework for centralized authorization of technical procedures for drugs in the European Union [16].
   - It establishes the role of the EMA, including the evaluation and monitoring of drugs and the decision-making process for marketing authorization.
2. Drug Evaluation Guidelines:
   - These guidelines provide information about drug testing and recommendations for behavior during drug development [17].
   - They introduce the principles of clinical trials, patient selection, evaluation of efficacy and safety, and statistical analysis.
3. Good Clinical Practice (GCP) Guidelines:
   - EMA's GCP Guidelines provide internationally recognized standards for the design, conduct, documentation, and reporting of clinical trials.
   - These guidelines help to ensure the protection of the rights, safety and health of the research participants and the reliability of the research results.
4. Guidelines for the Good Use of Medicines (GVP):
   - GVP guidelines provide a framework for the collection, management, and reporting of drug safety information.
   - They cover all aspects of pharmacovigilance, including reporting of adverse drug reactions, risk management, detection, and safety communication.
5. Pharmaceutical Quality Guidelines:
   - These guidelines address aspects of pharmaceutical quality, including pharmaceutical design, production, and management.
   - They indicate Good Manufacturing Practices for different types of drugs, such as chemical, biological, and herbal.

6. Biosimilars Guidance:
   - The EMA Biosimilars Guidance provides principles and guidelines for the development and licensing of biosimilars.
   - It provides guidance on information needed for comparative studies and validation showing similarity to biological materials used.

9.2.9 EMA's ROLE IN THE COVID-19 PANDEMIC

The EMA has played a key role in the response to the COVID-19 pandemic [18] by supporting the development, approval, and monitoring of vaccines and therapy.

An overview of EMA's role in the COVID-19 outbreak:

1. Rapid development and approval:
   - EMA has implemented a rapid process to facilitate rapid development and approval for safe and effective COVID-19 vaccines and treatments.
   - It provides scientific advice to pharmaceutical companies developing anti-COVID-19 drugs and treatments to improve their development plans and conduct robust clinical trials.
2. Regulatory marketing authorization:
   - The EMA has granted a Regulatory Marketing Authorization for a vaccine against COVID-19 based on available data showing it to be safe, effective, and of good quality.
   - This consent-based marketing authorization provides timely access to vaccines, while continuous data collection and monitoring are required to ensure that the benefit-risk balance remains favorable.
3. Continuous safety monitoring:
   - The EMA has established a strict pharmacovigilance unit to monitor the safety and efficacy of COVID-19 vaccines and treatment.
   - It works closely with national regulators and international partners to collect and analyze safety data and take appropriate regulatory action as needed.
4. Public health communications and information:
   - EMA provides transparent and timely communication to healthcare professionals, patients, and the public about COVID-19 vaccines and treatments [19].
   - It posts safety updates, product information, and recommendations on the use of COVID-19 vaccines and treatments on its website to ensure that the information is accurate and reliable.
5. International cooperation:
   - EMA cooperates with international regulatory bodies (e.g., USA).
   - The U.S. Food and Drug Administration and the World Health Organization share information and collaborate on regulatory approaches to COVID-19 vaccines and treatments.

- This collaboration can help to achieve harmonization of regulatory standards and support global access to safe and effective COVID-19 responses.

9.3 PHARMACEUTICAL INSPECTION CO-OPERATION SCHEME (PIC/S)

9.3.1 ORIGIN AND EVOLUTION

The Pharmaceutical Inspection Co-Operation Scheme (PIC/S) came into existence in 1995 as a development of the Pharmaceutical Inspection Convention (PIC) that was established in 1970 by the European Free Trade Association (EFTA) [20]. The creation of PIC/S emerged as an important step as before this scheme, only the countries that were members of the EFTA could participate in the PIC. Apart from this, there was also no provision for ensuring whether the participating countries were meeting the standards set by PIC. The scope of PIC/S was expanded to include medicinal products for human as well as veterinary use [21]. The standards or requirements cannot be enforced as it is not a legal authority, the participating countries, however, agree to implement them.

The efforts to harmonize GMP (Good Manufacturing Practice) standards for pharmaceutical products, have constantly been made ever since the inception of PIC/S. Several guidance documents and tools have also been developed to support the inspections like, the Site Master File (SMF) and the Recommendation on Quality System Requirements for Pharmaceutical Inspectorates.

In the recent past, PIC/S has actively promoted the concept of global GMP compliance [22]. The milestones in the evolution of PIC/S (Figure 9.3):

1970: establishment of PIC by EFTA (European Free Trade Association)
1995: foundation of PIC/S with expanded scopes and objectives
2001: first published GMP Guide based on the WHO GMP guide
2005: first published guidance document on the Site Master File (SMF)
2010: first published guidance document on the quality system requirements
2017: first published guidance document on the Manufacture of Active Pharmaceutical Ingredients (APIs)
2022: expansion of mandate to include GMP for medical devices.

9.3.2 MEMBERSHIP AND ORGANIZATIONAL FRAMEWORK

The process for getting a membership in PIC/S is discrete. Any regulatory authority having a similar GMP inspection system can become a member by submitting an application to the PIC/S Secretariat. The PIC/S Committee then reviews the application and only after acceptance, the authority will be considered a PIC/S Participating Authority (PA). At present, it has 54 Participating Authorities from all continents [23].

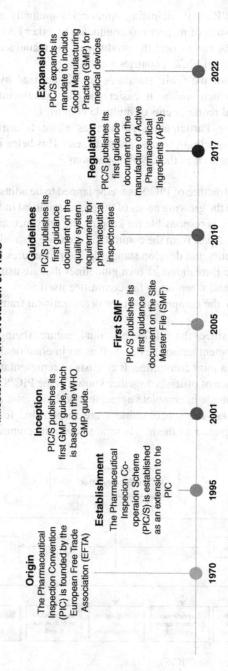

Milestones in the evolution of PIC/S

Origin
The Pharmaceutical Inspection Convention (PIC) is founded by the European Free Trade Association (EFTA)

1970

Establishment
The Pharmaceutical Inspection Co-operation Scheme (PIC/S) is established as an extension to he PIC

1995

Inception
PIC/S publishes its first GMP guide, which is based on the WHO GMP guide.

2001

First SMF
PIC/S publishes its first guidance document on the Site Master File (SMF)

2005

Guidelines
PIC/S publishes its first guidance document on the quality system requirements for pharmaceutical inspectorates

2010

Regulation
PIC/S publishes its first guidance document on the manufacture of Active Pharmaceutical Ingredients (APIs)

2017

Expansion
PIC/S expands its mandate to include Good Manufacturing Practice (GMP) for medical devices

2022

FIGURE 9.3 Milestones in evolution (PICS).

The following are the benefits of being a PIC/S Participating Authority:

- **Inspections:** PIC/S Participating Authorities mutually agree to take into account the results of inspections conducted by other PAs. This refers to the fact that any PA can inspect the products of the manufacturers and approve them for sale in all PIC/S countries.
- **Harmonization:** the GMP standards are harmonized by the Participating Authorities, which makes it easier for the manufacturers to fulfill the pharmaceutical requirements of multiple countries.
- **Exchange:** the Participating Authorities share information on various aspects like inspections, trends, practices, etc. This helps improve the safety of medicines as well as the GMP inspections.

The organizational structure of PIC/S is well-planned to be adjustable and effective so that it can adapt to the growing needs of the pharmaceutical industry (Figure 9.4). The PIC/S committee is responsible for keeping the relevance and effectiveness of the scheme in check. Apart from the committee, there are also other subcommittees that help PAs to discuss and develop standards and procedures in specific areas of GMP. The Executive Bureau has its own guidelines that are usually in compliance with the committee and it reports to the committee itself.

The following are the components of the organizational framework [24]:

- **Committee:** since the PIC/S has dual nature (being an arrangement between competent authorities as well as an international treaty), the PIC/S Committee is a joint committee. It consists of representatives from each PA and a committee of officials, together known as the PIC/S committee. All the decisions are made in complete agreement with the joint committee.
- **Subcommittees:** the subcommittees are responsible for specific areas of work as designated to them. There are seven subcommittees that help in

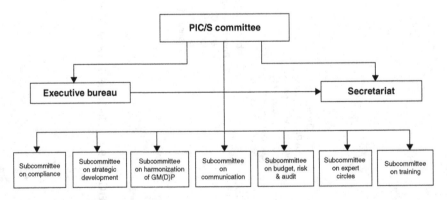

FIGURE 9.4 Organogram (PIC/S).

training, strategic development, risk management, and harmonization of GMP standards.

- **Executive Bureau:** it consists of the Chairperson, Deputy Chairperson, the immediate past Chairperson, the Chairs of the Subcommittees, and the Secretary. The bureau reports to the PIC/S committee.
- **Secretariat:** the secretariat is composed of a Secretary, a Deputy Secretary, a Treasurer, and an Assistant Secretary. All the staff is appointed by the executive bureau.

9.3.3 FOCUS AREAS

The main focus of the PIC/S is to provide improved public health by making sure that the GMP standards are being followed [25]. This is accomplished by the harmonization of GMP standards worldwide, mutual recognition of inspections, providing necessary training and networking between the PIC/S Authorities.

PIC/S cannot enforce its standards or procedures, as it is an autonomous organization. The standards and procedures are still widely accepted throughout the world, because of the benefits it has provided in protecting public health by improving the quality of pharmaceutical products.

PIC/S's work is important as it makes sure that the medicines meant for a person's well-being are safe and effective [26]. The ultimate goal remains the same, i.e., the protection of public health [27].

Apart from the core activities, PIC/S is also involved in other initiatives:

- Development of guidance documents on GMP and inspection procedures
- Research on GMP and inspection topics
- Use of information technology in GMP and inspection
- Developing GMP inspection capacity in economically developing nations

9.3.4 HARMONIZATION OF GMP STANDARDS

Harmonization of GMP standards and maintaining the quality systems of inspectorates are the main objectives of the PIC/S. These are fulfilled by adopting common GMP guidelines and executing a mutual recognition arrangement (MRA) for inspections.

The PIC/S GMP guide is an all-inclusive document that has all the requirements and standards for the manufacture of medicinal products [28]. This guide is based on the WHO GMP Guide with further developments in view of the PIC/S PAs. Additional guidance documents include the below [29]:

- The Site Master File
- Guidelines outlining the quality system requirements
- Guidelines for the manufacture of active pharmaceutical ingredients

All these documents help to ensure that the inspections are conducted in a consistent and harmonized manner.

Another important tool for the harmonization of GMP inspections is the MRA. It allows the PIC/S PAs to accept the results of inspections conducted by other MRA partners. This means that the inspection results will be acceptable to all MRA partners, while any MRA partner can inspect the manufacturers [30].

Benefits of harmonization by PIC/S are as follows:

- Increase in confidence in the quality of medicinal products
- Reduction in barriers to trade
- Efficient GMP inspections
- Worldwide harmonization of GMP requirements

9.3.5 EXCHANGE OF INFORMATION AND BEST PRACTICES

The exchange of information and best practices plays an important part in the organization's work ensuring the quality and safety of medicinal products manufactured in PIC/S partner countries. The exchange of information in PIC/S is typically bilateral, meaning it is between two PAs. There are some multilateral exchanges of information also, like those that take place through MRAs. The exchange of information is necessary for the performance of MRAs. To participate in an MRA, PAs must agree to the exchange of information on GMP inspections. The information includes the results of inspections along with the corrective and preventive actions if taken. Other modes of multilateral exchange of information are the PIC/S Electronic Exchange of Information (EEOI).

The benefits of this exchange of information and best practices are as follows:

- It ensures that the PAs are aware of the latest guidelines of GMP.
- It facilitates the mutual recognition of GMP inspections.
- It helps in improving the quality and safety of medicinal products manufactured in the PIC/S countries.

9.3.6 TRAINING AND CAPACITY BUILDING

For effective inspections, it is necessary to provide high-quality training and capacity-building opportunities to compliant inspectors. PIC/S ensures that the inspectors have the necessary skills and knowledge needed for the effective regulation of the pharmaceutical industry.

The various trainings offered by PIC/S are as follows:

- **Training Courses for New Inspectors:** these courses aim at training newly appointed inspectors with no previous experience in GMP inspection.

- **Train the Trainer Courses:** these courses are for experienced inspectors who want to become trainers.
- **Training for Auditors:** this training has been developed by PIC/S and EMA for auditors of the Joint Re-assessment Programme (JRP) and Joint Audit Programme (JAP).
- **Expert Circles:** these are the group meetings of experts, which regularly discuss various aspects of GMP.
- **API International Training Programme:** this training program consists of three segments, general training (for regulators and industry), advanced training (for regulators only), and question-answer for regulators and industry.
- **Joint Visits' Programme:** in this program, joint inspections are conducted by inspectors from different PIC/S countries.
- **Coached Inspections' Programme:** this program is specifically designed for new inspectors or those who want to enhance their inspection skills in a particular area.

9.3.7 PIC/S AND INTERNATIONAL COLLABORATIONS

PIC/S, in collaboration with several other organizations, promotes the GMP standards harmonization and improves the quality and safety of medicinal products [31]. Some of these organizations are as follows:

- **The World Health Organization (WHO):** it is a leading international organization in the field of public health. PIC/S in association with the WHO helps better the quality and safety of medicinal products.
- **The European Medicines Agency (EMA):** it is the European Union's agency for the evaluation of medicines. For the mutual recognition of inspections, these two agencies operate between the EU and PIC/S countries.
- **The International Conference of Harmonization of Technical Requirements for Registration of Pharmaceuticals for Human Use (ICH):** it is an international organization that deals with the harmonization of GMP standards for registration of pharmaceuticals. As the primary objective of PIC/S is also the same, this makes it an efficient collaboration.
- **The International Organization for Standardization (ISO):** it is the world's leading formulator of international standards. PIC/S and ISO work together to harmonize GMP standards with ISO standards.
- These partnerships are important for ensuring the quality and safety of pharmaceutical products.

9.4 CHALLENGES AND FUTURE PERSPECTIVES

9.4.1 REGULATORY CHALLENGES

9.4.1.1 Regulatory Challenges Faced by EMA

1. Brexit impact:
   - The UK's exit from the European Union (EU) has created challenges for the EMA, including the need to relocate leadership and change functions and resources [20].
   - Brexit has also had an impact on the EMA's regulatory processes, such as the evaluation and approval of drugs and coordination with national authorities.
2. Increased workload:
   - EMA faces increased workload due to increased license applications, amendments, and pharmacovigilance activities [2].
   - Progress on the job requires effective management of resources, skills, and processes to ensure effective and efficient regulation of medicines.
3. Rapid progress:
   - Advances in technology in the pharmaceutical industry are making it difficult for the EMA to update its regulatory and evaluation process.
   - New industries such as gene therapy, advanced medical devices (ATMPs), and health technologies must be regulated to ensure safety, effectiveness, and appropriate risk management.

9.4.1.2 REGULATORY CHALLENGES FACED BY PIC/S

1. Global Regulatory Convergence:
   - Regulatory convergence among PIC/S member countries is difficult to achieve due to differences in national regulations and practices [21].
   - Harmonization of Good Manufacturing Practice (GMP) standards and audit procedures requires continuous effort to ensure and improve compliance with quality standards.
2. The Changing Pharmaceutical Landscape:
   - The pharmaceutical industry is rapidly changing with new treatments, such as biologics, biosimilars, and personalized medicines.
   - Ensuring appropriate regulatory and review processes in emerging areas (such as complex biotechnology products) poses challenges for PIC/S.
3. Allocating resources and capacity building:
   - It is difficult for PIC/S to develop the capacity to review and increase the capacity of regulators, especially in developing countries.
   - Strengthening capacity building and assistance delivery is essential to support cohesion and reconciliation.

9.4.2 ADAPTATION TO TECHNOLOGICAL ADVANCEMENTS

Adaptation to technological developments is essential for effective monitoring of the pharmaceutical industry by regulatory bodies such as the European Medicines Agency (EMA) and the Pharmaceutical Inspection Co-Operation Program (PIC/S) [22]. The details of its transition to technological innovation are as follows:

EMA technological innovation:

1. Digitization of administrative processes:
   - EMA uses technology to simplify administrative processes and increase efficiency. This includes the use of electronic transmission systems for business licenses, medical records, and safety reports.
   - EMA is also exploring the use of advanced data science, artificial intelligence (AI), and machine learning to improve data analysis, signal analysis, and risk assessment [22].
2. Use of real-world evidence (RWE):
   - The EMA updates the use of real-world evidence in regulatory decision-making. RWE includes data from sources, such as electronic medical records, patient records, and clinical studies [23].
   - The EMA is developing guidelines and a framework to facilitate the use of RWE in the regulatory process, including post-authorization safety and effectiveness assessments [23].

Digital Health Technologies

- EMA collaborates with health technologies, such as mHealth applications, wearables, and telemedicine.
- It researches legal practices to ensure that health technologies are safe, effective, and protect personal information. It also develops mechanisms to evaluate and monitor health technologies [22].

PIC/S Adaptation to Technological Advances:

1. Updated Good Manufacturing Practice (GMP) Guidelines:
   - PIC/S regularly updates its GMP Guidelines to accommodate technological advances, such as output and production process design.
   - The new guidance sets clear expectations for the use of new technologies, such as improved production processes, automation, and quality control [21].
2. Audit of Quality Manufacturing Facilities:
   - PIC/S ensures that audit procedures and training include auditing of advanced manufacturing facilities, including continuous production and the use of new technologies, such as 3D printing.

- The aim is to evaluate the use of quality and risk management techniques related to this technology [21].
3. Education and Knowledge Exchange:
   - PIC/S organizes workshops, seminars, and conferences to promote knowledge sharing and best practices in technology developments.
   - These projects facilitate the sharing of learning among managers, facilitating cohesion and collaboration [21].

9.4.3 FUTURE DIRECTIONS AND INNOVATIONS

The European Medicines Agency (EMA) and the Pharmaceutical Inspection Co-Operation Program (PIC/S) are constantly evolving to meet future challenges and embrace new developments in the pharmaceutical industry. The following are the future directions and innovations of EMA and PIC/S:

Future directions of EMA:

1. Advanced therapy:
   - EMA's policies for new therapies, including advanced medical products (ATMPs), such as genes and cells, works to support therapy.
   - This includes the development of guidelines and the provision of scientific advice to support the development and regulatory approval of these treatments [24, 25].
2. Personalized medicine:
   - The EMA is also exploring the regulation of personalized medicine, i.e., tailoring of treatment to the patient's characteristics.
   - This includes deciding on specific guidelines and strategies for reviewing and authorizing personalized medicine [24].
3. Digital Health and Artificial Intelligence (AI):
   - EMA is involved in the new healthcare and intelligence business, which includes technologies such as healthcare applications, wearables, and AI-driven algorithms for drug discovery and development.
   - EMA ensures that these technologies are secure, efficient, and protect personal data.

Future Directions for PIC/S:
1. Strengthening harmonization:
   - PIC/S aims to strengthen the global regulatory framework and harmonize the GMP standards and audit procedures of member states and other regulatory bodies.
   - This includes promoting the integration of surveillance and supporting the review process.

2. Continuous capacity building:
    - PIC/S is committed to strengthening the analytical and regulatory capacity of its member institutions, particularly in developing countries.
    - This includes providing training, holding workshops, and facilitating the exchange of information to ensure global compliance with GMP standards.
3. New Manufacturing Technologies:
    - PIC/S adopts innovative manufacturing technologies, such as continuous manufacturing, 3D printing and process analytical technology (PAT).
    - Designed to develop guidance and assessment procedures to address specific and quality control issues related to this technology.

REFERENCES

1. EMA. European Medicines Agency: About Us. Available from www.ema.europa.eu/en/about-us/who-we-are.
2. EMA. European Medical Agency. Available from www.ema.europa.eu/en/about-us/who-we-are.
3. EMA. European Medicines Agency. Available from www.ema.europa.eu/en/about-us/what-we-do.
4. EMA. Marketing Authorization. Available from www.ema.europa.eu/en/human-regulatory/marketing-authorisation.
5. EMA. Pharmacovigilance: post-authorisation. Available from www.ema.europa.eu/en/human-regulatory/post-authorisation/pharmacovigilance-post-authorisation.
6. EMA. Human medicines: regulatory information. Available from www.ema.europa.eu/en/human-medicines-regulatory-information.
7. EMA. Guideline on the acceptability of names for human medicinal products processed through the centralised procedure - Scientific guideline. Available from www.ema.europa.eu/en/guideline-acceptability-names-human-medicinal-products-processed-through-centralised-procedure.
8. EMA. Scientific advice and protocol assistance. Available from www.ema.europa.eu/en/human-regulatory/research-development/scientific-advice-protocol-assistance.
9. EMA. Paediatric medicines: research and development. Available from www.ema.europa.eu/en/human-regulatory/research-development/paediatric-medicines-research-development.
10. EMA. Orphan designation: research and development. Available from www.ema.europa.eu/en/human-regulatory/research-development/orphan-designation-research-development.
11. EMA. International activities. Available from www.ema.europa.eu/en/partners-networks/international-activities.
12. EMA. International Affairs. Available from www.ema.europa.eu/en/documents/leaflet/international-cooperation-european-medicines-agency_en.pdf#:~:text=EMA%20has%20played%20an%20international%20role%20since%20its,well%20as%20collaboration%20with%20WHO%20on%20international%20pharmacovigilance.

13. EMA. International Council on Harmonisation of Technical Requirements for Registration of Pharmaceuticals for Human Use (ICH). Available from www.ema. europa.eu/en/partners-networks/international-activities/multilateral-coalitions-init iatives/international-council-harmonisation-technical-requirements-registration-pharmaceuticals-human-use.

14. EMA. International Coalition of Medicines Regulatory Authorities (ICMRA). Available from www.ema.europa.eu/en/partners-networks/international-activities/multilateral-coalitions-initiatives/international-coalition-medicines-regulatory-auth orities-icmra.

15. EDQM. Pharmacopoeial Harmonisation. Available from www.edqm.eu/en/pha rmacopoeial-harmonisation.

16. Commisssion E. Regulation (EC) No 726/2004 of the European Parliament and of the Council. Available from https://health.ec.europa.eu/system/files/2016-11/reg_2004_726_en_0.pdf.

17. EMA. Article 5 procedure: regulatory and procedural guidance. Available from www.ema.europa.eu/en/human-regulatory/post-authorisation/variations/article-5-procedure-regulatory-procedural-guidance.

18. EMA. Coronavirus disease (COVID-19). Available from www.ema.europa.eu/en/human-regulatory/overview/public-health-threats/coronavirus-disease-covid-19.

19. EMA. COVID-19 vaccines: development, evaluation, approval and monitoring. Available from www.ema.europa.eu/en/human-regulatory/overview/public-health-threats/coronavirus-disease-covid-19/covid-19-public-health-emergency-internatio nal-concern-2020-23/covid-19-vaccines-development-evaluation-approval-mon itoring.

20. EMA. Brexit: the United Kingdom's withdrawal from the European Union. Available from www.ema.europa.eu/en/about-us/history-ema/brexit-united-kingd oms-withdrawal-european-union.

21. PIC/S. Pharmaceutical Inspection Co-Operation Scheme. Available from https://picscheme.org/.

22. EMA. Questions and answers: qualification of digital technology-based methodologies to support approval of medicinal products 2020. Available from www.ema.europa.eu/en/documents/other/questions-answers-qualification-digital-technology-based-methodologies-support-approval-medicinal_en.pdf.

23. PIC/S. Use of real-world evidence in regulatory decision making – EMA publishes review of its studies 2023. Available from www.ema.europa.eu/en/news/use-real-world-evidence-regulatory-decision-making-ema-publishes-review-its-studies.

24. EMA. Innovation in medicines. Available from www.ema.europa.eu/en/human-reg ulatory/research-development/innovation-medicines.

25. EMA. Advanced therapies: research and development. Available from www.ema. europa.eu/en/human-regulatory/research-development/advanced-therapies-resea rch-development.

26. PIC/S. GMP oversight of medicines manufacturers in the European Union. Available from www.pda.org/pda-letter-portal/home/full-article/gmp-oversight-of-medicines-manufacturers-in-the-european-union.

27. PIC/S. Introduction. Available from picscheme.org/en/about-introduction.

28. PIC/S. Guide to good manufacturing practice for medicinal products annexes. 14 rue du Roveray CH-1207 Geneva2022.

29. PIC/S. Article – The 5 Ps of GMP. Available from www.vitafoodsinsights.com/lab-and-quality-control/5-ps-gmp.
30. PIC/S. Frequently asked questions. Available from https://picscheme.org/en/f-a-q.
31. PIC/S. PIC/S Inspectorates' Academy. Available from https://picscheme.org/en/pia-home.

10 Quality Control Considerations Specific to the Development and Production of Gene and Cell Therapies

Tara Chand and Ashwini Kumar Dubey
National Institute of Biologicals, Ministry of Health and
Family Welfare, Government of India, A-32, Sector-62,
Noida – 201309, India

10.1 BACKGROUND

The "cell and gene therapies" (CGTs) are also known as "regenerative medicines" or "advanced therapy medicinal products" (ATMPs). The CGTs include four types of therapies – gene therapies, gene modified cell therapies, cell therapies, and tissue engineered products (Figure 10.1). Unlike traditional biotech products, these therapies introduce cells and genes into a patient to treat the underlying cause of a disease or condition and providing a precision or personalized and targeted approach. Gene therapy is the modification or manipulation of the human or cellular genome to correct or replace defective genes [1] in order to treat inherited or acquired diseases while the cell therapy involves the transfer of live or intact cells in order to replace the damaged or diseased cells and to alter desired biological properties. The cells are modified outside the body and then delivered to the patients. Cell therapies has shown success in the treatment of solid tumors as well as blood cancers and hematological conditions, including lymphoma, leukaemia, and multiple myeloma. Stem cell therapies can treat spinal cord injuries, type I diabetes, Parkinson's disease, etc. In India, the "National Guidelines for Stem Cell Research 2017" [2] and "National Guidelines for Gene Therapy Product Development and Clinical Trials 2019" [3] describe the scientific and ethical considerations for the development and production of cell and gene therapy products and their therapeutic use. These guidelines also describe the quality control and quality assurance standards as well as the planning and conduct of preclinical and clinical trials. Today, a number of CGT products are developed

DOI: 10.1201/9781032697444-10

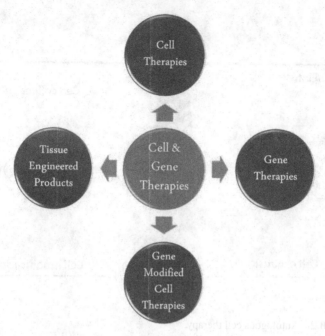

FIGURE 10.1   Types of cell and gene therapies.

and approved and several others are under clinical trials and we hope to see more life-saving and life-improving treatments to come. The quality attributes define the safety, purity, potency, identity, and stability of the CGT products. Hence, the quality of these products must be ensured by manufacturers at the production level as well as by the regulatory bodies before reaching the market to safeguard the public health [4]. This chapter aims to explore the various aspects of QC in gene and cell therapies, including the methods and technologies employed, the regulatory landscape, and the future directions in this rapidly evolving field.

10.2   CELL AND GENE THERAPY

10.2.1   PRODUCTION

The production of CGT products involves several key steps, including cell sourcing, genetic modification (in the case of gene therapies), cell expansion or manipulation, formulation, and final product testing. The cell sourcing begins with the collection of cells from a donor (allogeneic) or from the patient (autologous). Autologous therapies involve harvesting cells from the patient (Figure 10.2), typically from the blood, bone marrow, or solid tissue. Allogeneic therapies use cells from a healthy donor (Figure 10.3), often selected based on HLA matching. Once collected, the desired cell population is isolated and purified from the

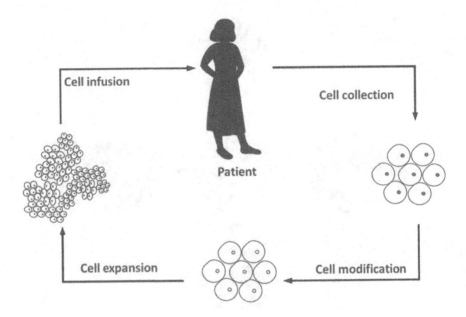

FIGURE 10.2   Autologous cell therapy.

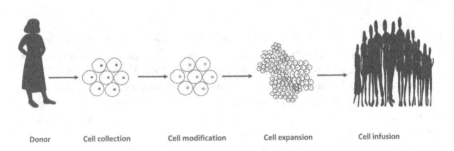

FIGURE 10.3   Allogenic cell therapy.

harvested sample [2, 5]. This step ensures that the appropriate cell type is obtained and removes unwanted cells or contaminants. In gene therapies, the isolated cells undergo genetic modification to introduce or modify specific genes [6]. This is typically done using viral vectors such as "lentiviral or adenoviral" vectors or non-viral systems such as "CRISPR-Cas9 technology or electroporation" [3]. The gene modification step aims to confer the desired therapeutic properties to the cells. The modified cells are then cultured and expanded to increase their numbers in the presence of appropriate growth factors, cytokines, and culture conditions essential for supporting the cell proliferation while maintaining their desired characteristics. After the desired cell population is obtained, it is formulated and prepared for administration to the patient. The final product is packaged in appropriate containers, such as cryovials or infusion bags. The cell therapies are cryopreserved using appropriate cryoprotective agents for long-term storage.

Like other biotherapeutics, the CGT products are subject to quality control (QC) testing, which includes testing for identity, potency, purity, endotoxin levels, sterility, mycoplasma contamination, and viral safety to safeguard the public health. A number of various molecular, immunological, and other analytical techniques, such as flow cytometry, etc., are employed to assess the product's characteristics and performance. The QC passed CGT products are released into marked for commercialization or distributed to hospital or clinical site for patients.

Compliance with Good Manufacturing Practices (GMP) and quality management systems during the entire production steps is critical for ensuring uniformity, reproducibility, safety, and other quality standards [2, 3]. Validation of the production processes, documentation, and regular monitoring are vital to ensure the product integrity [7]. The production process varies depending upon the type of CGT, the targeted disease, and the regulatory requirements of the country concerned.

10.2.2 Good Manufacturing Practice (GMP) Requirements

The GMP guidelines are essential to ensure the quality of CGT products and it emphasizes regular monitoring and documentation as well. GMP regulations require the design, construction, and maintenance of products to maintain appropriate environmental conditions, cleanliness, and contamination control, which may vary from country to country or location. It is important that sufficient space, equipment, and resources used to support production and ensure the quality of the final product and safety commodity. Furthermore, GMP mandates that tools and equipment used for CGTs must be periodically evaluated and maintained, which is suitable for intended users [2, 3]. A calibration tool, qualifications, and certification program are necessary to demonstrate the reliability, precision, and accuracy of the equipment. GMP regulations train and qualify personnel involved in manufacturing and quality control. Employees must be properly trained, competent, follow standard operating procedures (SOPs), and have the necessary knowledge and skills to perform their jobs effectively. The inspection process includes design procedures, key elements, qualification of tools and equipment, and ongoing inspection and control. GMP regulations govern the control of cellular and genetic materials. This includes developing specifications, testing for identification, purity and potency, as well as storage, transport, and inspection procedures to prevent contamination or damage [8].

GMP emphasizes the need for effective quality control systems and testing procedures to ensure the production, purity, safety, and quality of cell-gene therapy products. This includes using correct testing methods, establishing guidelines for product releases, and thoroughly testing finished products prior to their availability for use in clinical settings. In addition, GMP regulations require record keeping and proper documentation procedures. This includes accurate and current construction performance records, test findings, deviations, inspections, and corrective actions. Regulatory authorities should have controlled documentation that can be easily searched. Traceability and traceability systems must be maintained in accordance with GMP throughout the manufacturing process. It is part of the raw materials used, how they are converted into finished products, how they are used and distributed. When needed, these methods allow for process recalls and facilitate the identification and resolution of quality problems. GMP standards emphasize the importance of adopting change control procedures to monitor and document changes in processes, equipment, or raw materials. It must be properly tested, approved, and reported to ensure that the changes do not jeopardize the quality, safety, or efficacy of the product [2, 3]. GMP mandates internal repeat audits and regulatory monitoring to ensure compliance. Manufacturers should have systems in place to facilitate audits and inspections, including access to inspectors and critical information in their facilities [8].

The aforementioned GMP standards are designed to create a robust quality control system to assure safety, effectiveness, and quality. For CGT products to comply with regulations, manufacturers must keep pace with GMP standards and relevant regional regulations.

10.2.3 MANUFACTURING AND QUALIFICATION CHALLENGES

Because of their complexity and tailored approach, manufacturing and validation of cell and gene treatments face distinct obstacles. Patient-specific starting materials, such as autologous cells or personalized genetic constructs, are frequently used in cell and gene therapies [2, 3]. This heterogeneity complicates standardization because each patient's cells or genetic material may differ in quality and performance. Cell and gene therapies are often performed on a small number of patients and necessitate sophisticated manufacturing techniques. It might be difficult to scale up these procedures to suit commercial needs while preserving product quality and uniformity. Continuous difficulties include developing scalable manufacturing platforms and optimizing production efficiency [9]. It takes a lot of effort and time to develop and refine manufacturing procedures for cell and gene treatments. To ensure cell viability, genetic integrity, and product quality, process variables must be carefully regulated [7]. Due to the distinctive properties of many cell types and genetic constructs, determining the best growth conditions, gene delivery strategies, and purification approaches is difficult.

The handling and transportation of sensitive live cells, vectors, and other materials under strict temperature and time restrictions are part of the supply chain for cell and gene treatments. To preserve product viability and integrity, a strong and validated supply chain, including cold chain management, is essential.

In the manufacture of cell and gene therapies, as was previously noted, assuring product quality and safety presents substantial difficulties. Given that these treatments are highly customized, developing suitable quality control tests and release testing techniques can be challenging. It continues to be difficult to validate and implement these tests to accurately evaluate the consistency and quality of the produced products [9]. The regulatory landscape is constantly changing, making it difficult to stay on top of it when it comes to cell and gene treatments. In order to manufacture, regulate quality, and release these therapies in compliance with regulatory standards, it is necessary to have a thorough awareness of the relevant regulations and to be proactive in interacting with regulatory authorities.

Due to the vulnerability of live cells or genetic constructs to environmental conditions, cell and gene therapies frequently have poor stability and a short shelf life [7]. A big difficulty is figuring out the best storage settings and developing trustworthy stability testing procedures to guarantee product potency and efficacy throughout time. Cell and gene therapies are highly individualized, and their intricate manufacturing procedures sometimes lead to high manufacturing costs [10]. The broad use and accessibility of these medicines face difficulties in achieving cost-effective production and striking a balance between affordability, quality, and scalability [9].

Collaboration amongst stakeholders, such as researchers, clinicians, manufacturers, regulators, and patients, is necessary to address these issues. To get around these and make it easier to create, manufacture, and qualify cell and gene therapies, more innovation, technological improvements, and interdisciplinary work are required.

10.2.4 Automation in Cell and Gene Therapy

It is vital to emphasize that cell treatments are "living pharmaceuticals," which will necessitate modified, fit-for-purpose manufacturing techniques to address difficulties, such as inherent donor unpredictability, cell heterogeneity, insufficient scalability, and batch to batch inconsistencies.

There is a growing and urgent demand for industrial translation as more and more cell and gene treatments are being created and as more and more applications for regulatory approval are being made. Before cell and gene therapies may be industrialized, problems with process effectiveness, related cost drivers, and regulatory requirements must be resolved. These problems could be resolved by automation, which would also open the door to commercialization and mass production, as it did in the past for "classical" manufacturing industries [11, 12].

When it comes to allogenic "off-the-shell" medicines, in particular, automation can be crucial to scaling up manufacturing. Many of these current problems could be solved by automation without sacrificing the efficacy and safety of these treatments. Production automation is a crucial strategy to address quality, cost of products, scalability, and sustainability, which are basic drivers for economically viable production. It is both highly enticing and very complex at the same time [13]. At medical academic institutions, numerous production techniques are being developed but they lack the resources or the know-how to automate them. These academic institutions stand to gain from forming alliances with businesses that excel at integrating automation into production processes, such as pharmaceutical firms that have automated their processes, or organizations that have automated their processes.

The well-established biomanufacturing industries (such as biologics, monoclonal antibodies, small molecules, etc.) have shown that reducing manual labor time through automation provides a means of lowering human error, obtaining more repeatable results, achieving standardization, and enhancing the essential quality attributes of the finished product. These advantages might be attained through the automation of a single step, numerous automated steps, a workflow, or entirely automated work flows [14, 15]. Fully automated platforms would ideally provide an end-to-end solution from donor to product with continuous validation and monitoring for continuing process optimization operations. To lessen the possibility of contamination and human error, these devices could be completely closed, removing user touch. Unfortunately, the adaptability and flexibility needed for CGT applications are lacking in automation platforms made for biologics and monoclonal antibodies [14]. The industrial sector is currently experiencing the emergence of platforms that combine bioreactor and scaffold technologies to give total automation for both adherent and suspension cell cultures as part of ongoing efforts to increase automation [14]. The next stage for system developers is to recognize various elements that improve a bioprocessing approach and incorporate these into their work processes [4]. The distinction between allogenic and autologous therapy must be examined while considering CGT. Autologous therapies can benefit from a decentralized or hybrid approach, but allogenic therapies are compatible with centralized manufacturing, which is easier to scale up and reduces the initial investment in automation systems [15].

The complicated manufacturing process behind cell treatments makes them exceedingly pricey. Even while automation has the potential to decrease expenses in the long run, setting up automation and robotics can be highly expensive. Cell therapy production currently takes place on a number of different platforms, each of which has its own unique set of requirements. Due to a lack of uniformity, automating each of them would be expensive.

10.3   QUALITY CONTROL IN CELL AND GENE THERAPY

Quality control (QC) testing is an essential regulatory criterion that ensures that any cell or gene therapy provided is safe, effective, and meets a prescribed set of quality requirements. The CGT product must be rigorously evaluated to ensure that it remains effective during its designated shelf life before its clinical application. Analytical tests, as well as the equipment utilized in such tests, must be validated in compliance with stringent regulatory criteria. The QC testing protocols are updated from time to time when new technologies emerge [16]. The manufacturers must adhere to the regulatory guidelines issued by EMA or FDA or other as applicable in the country of origin. Such guidelines, ensure that the CGT products are safe and effective. Besides these, traceability should be there for tracking the CGT products throughout their lifecycles [17–19].

## 10.3.1	Testing Parameters

If the raw material is not pure and safe then the finished product will not be pure and safe. Hence, the testing of raw materials used in production of CGT products is vital to ensure the quality, safety, and potency of finished products. The testing parameters include analysis of purity, potency, sterility, safety, and stability, etc. These tests detect any impurities, microbial contaminations, pollutants, or other adulterations that affect the quality of the product and are a threat to the public health.

### 10.3.1.1	Purity and Microbiological Sterility

In the production of CGTs, the use of appropriate cell type or genetic material is a must. The raw materials used must be devoid of any microbial or other contamination [17–19]. Since, the cell-based therapies, due to their live nature, cannot be sterilized and therefore, sterility testing is necessary to ensure that there is no viral, bacterial, fungal, or mycoplasma contaminations [17–20]. Several techniques exist for the identification of microbial contaminations, rapid qPCR is one that sows particular promise.

The short tandem repeats (STR), which are 2–6 base pairs in length, is used to evaluate repeated segments of DNA. STR genotyping is used in routine authentication of cells and tissues as well as in the discrimination among DNA profiles. Karyotype analysis is used to detect culture-driven mutations, gross genetic alterations, duplications, deletions, inversions, or translocations.

The evaluation of the genetic material involve identification of the vector integration site, confirmation of proper expression of transgene and screening for potential genetic changes or mutations [20, 21]. Cutting-edge analytical methods like gene expression profiling, flow cytometry, proteomics, qPCR, or next-generation sequencing, etc., are employed to ensure the purity and identity of CGT products and raw materials used in its production [17, 18].

### 10.3.1.2	Potency

The assessment of cell viability and its functionality is essential to ensure intended biotherapeutic effects. A variety of tests can be used to evaluate particular characteristics like cell proliferation, cytokine release, or target cell death [19].

### 10.3.1.3	Safety

The human embryonic cells are capable of renewing and differentiating in to cells of the three germ layers. These traits make them tumorigenic too. Both in vivo and in vitro tests are employed to assess tumorigenicity of cryotherapies.

The immunocompromised animal models are used in the in vivo assessment of tumorigenicity of cryotherapies. The in vitro tests include cell proliferation assay, flow cytometry, karyotype analysis, qPCR, NGS, fluorescent in situ hybridization, etc.

10.3.1.4 Stability

The evaluation of stability involves the assessment of CGTs over time and in different environmental conditions, such as temperature, light, etc. Under these conditions the CGT product's shelf life and its integrity is calculated [17–19].

The QC testing parameters varies depending upon the type of CGT product, raw materials used, and regional regulatory requirements in the area where the CGT is being produced.

10.3.2 CONSEQUENCES OF SUBSTANDARD OR ADULTERATED PRODUCTS

It is crucial that manufacturers, researchers, and regulators prioritize and enforce robust quality control procedures, adhere to GMP guidelines, and conduct extensive preclinical and clinical testing to ensure the safety, efficacy, and quality of CGT products. Substandard products may fail to provide the intended treatment or may even harm patients. Inadequate quality control can lead to the contaminants, such as bacteria, viruses, or impurities, which can pose serious health risks. Additionally, if the therapy does not meet the required potency or functionality, it may not provide the expected clinical benefit to patients. This can lead to a lack of therapeutic response, disease progression, or inadequate symptom relief. Ineffective treatment can lead to prolonged suffering and reduced quality of life for patients.

Moreover, the substandard products can tarnish the reputation of the manufacturer, healthcare providers, and the field of regenerative medicine as a whole. Public confidence in these therapies can be undermined, leading to skepticism and reluctance among patients, healthcare professionals, and regulatory authorities. Rebuilding trust and confidence can be challenging and may impede future advancements in the field. Substandard products can lead to regulatory action, including product recalls, warning letters, or even the suspension or revocation of manufacturing licenses. Regulatory agencies may impose penalties or fines on manufacturers who fail to comply with quality standards. Additionally, patients who suffer harm as a result of substandard products may pursue legal actions against the manufacturer, leading to potential legal and financial consequences.

Substandard CGTs can hinder progress in the field of regenerative medicinal drug. If products fail to fulfill regulatory standards or exhibit significant safety or efficacy, it is able to affect the advancement of revolutionary treatment plans and obstruct the development of latest remedies. This can result in delays in bringing promising cures to patients and limit future research possibilities.

Developing and producing CGT products requires great investments of time, money, and expertise. If a product is substandard and cannot be used clinically, it is able to bring about wasted sources, including studies and improvement efforts, production costs, and medical trial costs. This can delay development within the subject and avert the provision of powerful therapies.

10.4   SALIENT APPROVED CELL AND GENE THERAPY PRODUCTS

The development of CGTs is advancing. Over 2000 clinical trials are currently underway around the world, with over 200 in phase III. Over a dozen novel cell or gene therapies could be licensed for use in the United States, Europe, or both by the end of 2023 [22]. However, a number of CGT products are approved by US-FDA [23] and EMA [24] for their therapeutic use (Table 10.1). In countries, viz., China, New Zealand, Australia, Japan, Canada, South Korea several other CGTs have been approved for its marketing. In India, the CDSCO (Central Drugs Standard Control Organization) has given marketing authorization to CGT products, viz., Stempeucel (Stempeutics Research), Apceden (APAC Biotech), Ossgrow (RMS Regrow) & Cartigrow (RMS Regrow) [24].

10.5   FUTURE PERSPECTIVES OF REGULATION

CGT has the potential to revolutionize the treatment of various diseases, offering personalized and targeted treatment solutions. As this groundbreaking medical technology continues to evolve, ensuring that it is used safely and effectively is of utmost importance. Future strategies for CGT compliance highlight the challenges and opportunities ahead. It explores the key considerations of regulators, manufacturers, industry stakeholders, and pharmaceutical professionals in the context of rapidly evolving science and technology [65].

10.5.1   CHALLENGES IN REGULATION OF CGTs

As the characteristics of the CGT are complex and its development depends on rapidly advancing scientific and technological developments, its legislation poses many challenges. It requires that regulatory bodies must keep in touch with cutting-edge technologies and ensure that an appropriate framework is in place for dealing with emerging CGTs and their unique characteristics [66]. CGTs are usually standardized or individualized treatments, so these require legislative amendments to allow for changes in sources, processes, and treatment methods, to be established. Acts authorizing treatment that are perfectly designed while balancing and ensuring quality, capacity, safety, and effectiveness is a challenge

The complexity and diversity of the structure of the CGT adds to the complexity of the law. Establishing consistent standards for manufacturing, processing, and QC while allowing for customization and innovation is challenging. Developing robust QC methods that can reliably measure CGT detection, purity, potency, safety, and stability is an ongoing challenge.

TABLE 10.1
Approved Cell and Gene Therapy Products

S. No.	Product Type	Name of Product and Manufacturer	Description/Target	USFDA Approved Year	EMA Approved Year	References
1.	Gene Therapy	**Roctavian (Valactocogene roxaparovac)** Biomarin Pharmaceutical Inc.	Hemophilia A in adults	2023	2022	[25, 26]
2.	Gene Therapy	**Zynteglo (Betibeglogene autotemcel)** Bluebird bio, Inc., USA	*beta*-thalassemia in adult and pediatric patients	2022	2019	[27, 28]
3.	Gene Therapy	**Adstiladrin (nadofaragene firadenovec-vncg)** Ferring Pharmaceuticals, Switzerland	non-muscle-invasive bladder cancer	2022	---	[29]
4.	Cell Therapy (autologous, modified)	**Carrykti (ciltacabtagene autoleucel)** Janssen (Johnson & Johnson) Biotech Inc., Belgium	Relapsed or refractory multiple myeloma	2022	2022	[30, 31]
5.	Gene Therapy	**Hemgenix (etranacogene dezaparvovec)** CSL Behring, USA	Certain kinds of Hemophilia B	2022	2022	[32, 33]
6.	Gene Therapy	**Skysona (elivaldogene autotemcel)** Bluebird bio, Inc., USA	Cerebral adrenoleukodystrophy	2022	2021	[34, 35]

No.	Type	Product (Company)	Indication	Year	Year	References
7.	Cell Therapy (Allogenic)	**Stratagraft (cultured keratinocytes and dermal fibroblasts in murine collagen-dsat)** Stratatech corporation	Adults with thermal burns	2021	---	[36]
8.	Cell Therapy (Allogenic)	**Rethymic (allogeneic processed thymus tissue)** Enzyvant Therapeutics GmbH	Congenital athymia	2021	---	[37]
9.	Cell Therapy (Autologous modified)	**Breyanzi (lisocabtagene maraleucel)** Juno Therapeutics Inc., a Bristol-Myers Squibb Company	Large B-cell lymphoma	2022	2022	[38, 39]
10.	Cell-based Gene therapy	**Abecma (idecabtagene vicleucel)** Celgene Corporation, a Bristol-Myers Squibb Company	Multiple myeloma	2021	2021	[40, 41]
11.	Cell (Autologous, modified)	**Tecartus (brexucabtagene autoleucel)** Kite Pharma, Inc.	Relapsed or refractory mantle cell lymphoma	2021	2020	[42, 43]
12.	Gene Therapy	**Zolgensma (onasemnogene abeparvovec)** Novartis Gene Therapies, Inc.	Spinal Muscular Atropy (Type I)	2019	2020	[44, 45]
13.	Cell Therapy	**HPC Cord Blood** MD Anderson Cord blood bank	Hematopoietic disorders	2018	---	[46]
14.	Gene Therapy	**Yescarta (axicabtagene ciloleucel)** Kite Pharma, Inc.	B-cell lymphoma	2017	2017	[47, 48]

(continued)

TABLE 10.1 (Continued)
Approved Cell and Gene Therapy Products

S. No.	Product Type	Name of Product and Manufacturer	Description/Target	USFDA Approved Year	EMA Approved Year	References
15.	Gene Therapy	**Luxturna (voretigene neparvovec)** Spark Therapeutics, Inc.	Biallelic RPE65 mutation-associated retinal dystrophy	2017	2018	[49, 50]
16.	Gene Therapy	**Kymriah (tisagenlecleucel)** Novartis Pharmaceuticals Corporation	Relapsed or refractory follicular lymphoma	2017	2017	[51, 52]
17.	Cell Therapy	**Clevecord** Cleveland Cord Blood Center	Hematopoietic disorders	2016	---	[53]
18.	Cell Therapy	**HPC Cord Blood** Life South Community Blood Centers, Inc.	Hematopoietic disorders	2016	---	[54]
19.	Cell Therapy	**HPC Cord Blood** Bloodworks	Hematopoietic disorders	2016	---	[55]
20.	Tissue Engineered Product	**Maci (Autologous Cultured Chondrocytes)** Vericel Corp.	Single or multiple symptomatic, full-thickness cartilage defects of the knee	2016	---	[56]
21.	Gene Therapy	**Imlygic (Talimogene laherparepvec)** Biovax, Inc., a subsidiary of Amgen Inc.	Unresectable cutaneous, subcutaneous, and nodal lesions	2015	---	[57]

22.	Cell Therapy	Allocord SSM Cardinal Glennon Children's Medical Center	Hematopoietic disorders	2013	[58]
23.	Cell Therapy	HPC, Cord Blood Cliniimmune Labs, University of Colorado Cord Blood Bank	Hematopoietic disorders	2012	[59]
24.	Cell Therapy	Ducord (HPC Cord Blood) Duke University, School of Medicine	Hematopoietic disorders	2012	[60]
26.	Tissue Engineered Product	Gintuit (Allogeneic Cultured Keratinocytes and Fibroblasts in Bovine Collagen) Organogenesis, Inc.	Mucogingival conditions	2012	[61]
27.	Cell Therapy	Hemacord New York Blood Center	Hematopoietic disorders	2011	[62]
28.	Cell Therapy	Laviv (Azficel-T) Fibrocell Technologies	Nasolabial fold wrinkles	2011	[63]
29.	Cell Therapy	Provenge (sipuleucel-T) Dendreon Corp.	Metastatic castrate resistant (hormone refractory) prostate cancer	2010	[64]

Furthermore, it is also important to ensure that regulatory agencies have the necessary skills and resources to successfully evaluate these treatments if they are to build regulatory capacity, with mandated oversight bodies, researchers, industry, and an intervention among others is a challenge in the rapidly developing field of regenerative medicine [65–67].

10.5.2 GLOBAL HARMONIZATION OF REGULATORY STANDARDS

CGT products are regulated by regulatory bodies around the world. Legal systems vary from country to country or region to region. Legal standards for CGT are very difficult to harmonize globally due to differences in legal guidelines and terminology. Global cooperation between regulatory bodies becomes important if global harmonization and CGT legal standards will be simplified. This will enable knowledge sharing, and accelerate the development and availability of CGTs across jurisdictions [65].

The "International Collaborative Council on Technical Requirements for Medicinal Products (ICH)" brings together regulatory agencies and pharmaceutical companies to discuss and cooperate on research related to drug development, registration, and licensing around [68]. The ICH's goal is to improve public health by harmonizing criteria and procedures for drug licensing for mutual benefit [67, 69].

10.5.3 FUTURE REGULATORY STRATEGIES AND INNOVATIONS

As CGT business processes improve, regulatory bodies' approaches to ensuring quality, consistency, and safety will continue. Adding optimization technologies, implementing comprehensive quality assurance inspections and programs, and reviewing standards can all be part of this. To accommodate the unique characteristics of these medicines, such as standardized and patient-specific therapy, there may be changes to better and more flexible regulation. Regulatory authorities may seek alternative ways to dispense medicines that have safe and effective manufacturing and rapid licensing while maintaining the critical patient safety standards [65]. Regulatory agencies are taking a more risk-based regulatory approach, focusing resources and inspections on high-risk chemicals and areas of concern. These policies may include unique requirements based on specific characteristics of various drugs, such as type of genetic modification, targeted disease, or intended patient population. This allows for sophisticated and harmonized CGT products [67].

Given the complexity of CGTs, regulatory bodies prioritize education and training for its staff, academics, physicians, and industry professionals. This leads to a better understanding of the scientific, technological, and legal aspects of these products, leading to more effective regulation, compliance, and communication between stakeholders.

10.5.4 POST-MARKETING SURVEILLANCE

In addition to clinical trials, it is important to monitor the safety and long-term efficacy of CGT drugs. Regulatory authorities face obstacles in developing post-marketing surveillance programs and long-term follow-up to assess the sustainability of responses, potential long-term adverse effects, and actual outcomes in the 21st century [70, 71]. States should develop national regulations and procedures for the post-marketing surveillance of biomaterials in phase IV clinical trials (Drugs and Cosmetics Act). Physicians, and healthcare providers, should be strongly encouraged to report any unexpected adverse effects that occur to patients after using these products to state regulators and the manufacturer.

The future of gene and cell therapies will be defined through continuous improvement of quality, collaboration, and patient-centered approaches. Regulators seek to strike a balance between innovation and patient safety, providing faster patient access to safe and effective medicines while promising careful monitoring and evaluation throughout the product lifecycle. Continued regulatory review and reform, harmonization efforts, and active participation of the scientific and medical communities are essential to promote safe production, research, and availability of CGT products and effectiveness encouraged.

REFERENCES

1. USFDA. What is Gene Therapy? US FDA. Available from www.fda.gov/vaccines-blood-biologics/cellular-gene-therapy-products/what-gene-therapy.
2. ICMR, DBT. National Guidelines for Stem Cell Research. ICMR, New Delhi; 2017.
3. ICMR, CDSCO, DBT. National Guideline for Gene Therapy Product Development & Clinical Trails. ICMR, New Delhi; 2019.
4. Ball O, Robinson S, Bure K, Brindley DA, Mccall D. Bioprocessing automation in cell therapy manufacturing: outcomes of special interest group automation workshop. Cytotherapy. 2018;20(4):592–9.
5. Hall V. Porcine embryonic stem cells: a possible source for cell replacement therapy. Stem Cell Reviews. 2008;4(4):275–82.
6. Anderson WF. Human gene therapy. Nature. 1998;392(4025):25–30.
7. Campbell A, Brieva T, Raviv L, Rowley J, Niss K, Brandwein H, et al. Concise review: process development considerations for cell therapy. Stem Cells Translational Medicine. 2015;4(10):1155–63.
8. Averall K. Cell and Gene Therapies & Their GMP Requirements. Available from https://ispe.org/pharmaceutical-engineering/cell-gene-therapies-their-gmp-requirements.
9. Bhattacharya S, Telang A. Manufacturing and Qualification Challenges for Cell and Gene Therapy Products and Best Practices for Success. Available from https://cellculturedish.com/manufacturing-and-qualification-challenges-for-cell-and-gene-therapy-products-and-best-practices-for-success/.
10. MacDonald A, Whelan S. Cell and Gene Therapy: Current Challenges and the Benefits of Automation. Available from www.technologynetworks.com/biopharma/blog/cell-and-gene-therapy-current-challenges-and-the-benefits-of-automation-367167.

11. Moutsatsou P, Ochs J, Schmitt RH, Hewitt CJ, Hanga MP. Automation in cell and gene therapy manufacturing: from past to future. Biotechnology Letters. 2019;41(11):1245–53.

12. Markarian J. Automation Aids Cell and Gene Therapy Production. Available from www.pharmtech.com/view/automation-aids-cell-and-gene-therapy-production.

13. Smith D, Heathman TRJ, Klarer A, LeBlon C, Tada Y, Hampson B. Towards automated manufacturing for cell therapies. Current Hematologic Malignancy Reports. 2019;14(4):278–85.

14. Spielvogel C, Stoiber S, Papp L, Krajnc D, Grahovac M, Gurnhofer E, et al. Radiogenomic markers enable risk stratification and inference of mutational pathway states in head and neck cancer. European Journal of Nuclear Medicine and Molecular Imaging. 2023;50:546–58.

15. Events R. Automation is key in cell and gene therapy manufacturing. Available from www.reutersevents.com/pharma/clinical/automation-key-cell-and-gene-therapy-manufacturing.

16. CCRM. Planning Is Everything - Quality Control Testing in Cell and Gene Therapy. Available from https://cdmo.ccrm.ca/blog/compendial-quality-control-testing-in-cell-and-gene-therapy.

17. Trott M. Key Techniques in Cell Therapy Quality Control. Available from www.technologynetworks.com/biopharma/lists/key-techniques-in-cell-therapy-quality-control-331890.

18. Sullivan S, Stacey G, Akazawa C, Aoyama N, Baptista R, Bedford P, et al. Quality control guidelines for clinical-grade human induced pluripotent stem cell lines. Regenerative Medicine. 2018;13(7):859–66.

19. Catapult CGT. Quality control in cell and gene therapy manufacturing Available from https://ct.catapult.org.uk/news/quality-control-in-cell-and-gene-therapy-manufacturing.

20. Li Y, Huo Y, Yu L, Wang J. Quality control and nonclinical research on CAR-T cell products: general principles and key issues. Engineering 2019;5(1):122–31.

21. Macdonald GJ. Gene therapy production and quality control. Available from www.genengnews.com/news/gene-therapy-production-and-quality-control/.

22. Hunt T. The cell and gene therapy sector in 2023: a wave is coming – are we ready? Available from https://invivo.pharmaintelligence.informa.com/IV146781/The-Cell-And-Gene-Therapy-Sector-In-2023-A-Wave-Is-Coming--Are-We-Ready.

23. USFDA. Approved Cellular and Gene Therapy Products. Available from www.fda.gov/vaccines-blood-biologics/cellular-gene-therapy-products/approved-cellular-and-gene-therapy-products.

24. ISCT. Cell, Tissue and Gene Products with Marketing Authorization. Available from www.isct-unprovencellulartherapies.org/68-2/.

25. Biomarin. U.S. Food and Drug Administration Approves BioMarin's ROCTAVIAN™ (valoctocogene roxaparvovec-rvox), the First and Only Gene Therapy for Adults with Severe Hemophilia A 2023. Available from https://investors.biomarin.com/2023-06-29-U-S-Food-and-Drug-Administration-Approves-BioMarins-ROCTAVIAN-TM-valoctocogene-roxaparvovec-rvox-,-the-First-and-Only-Gene-Therapy-for-Adults-with-Severe-Hemophilia-A.

26. Biomarin. First Gene Therapy for Adults with Severe Hemophilia A, BioMarin's ROCTAVIAN™ (valoctocogene roxaparvovec), Approved by European Commission

(EC) 2023b. Available from https://investors.biomarin.com/2022-08-24-First-Gene-Therapy-for-Adults-with-Severe-Hemophilia-A,-BioMarins-ROCTAVIAN-TM-valoctocogene-roxaparvovec-,-Approved-by-European-Commission-EC.

27. USFDA. FDA Approves First Cell-Based Gene Therapy to Treat Adult and Pediatric Patients with Beta-thalassemia Who Require Regular Blood Transfusions 2022. Available from www.fda.gov/news-events/press-announcements/fda-appro ves-first-cell-based-gene-therapy-treat-adult-and-pediatric-patients-beta-thalasse mia-who.

28. EMA. ZYNTEGLO: Autorization Details 2019. Available from www.ema.europa. eu/en/medicines/human/EPAR/zynteglo#authorisation-details-section.

29. USFDA. FDA D.I.S.C.O. Burst Edition: FDA approval of Adstiladrin (nadofaragene firadenovec-vncg) for patients with high-risk Bacillus Calmette-Guérin unresponsive non-muscle invasive bladder cancer with carcinoma in situ with or without papillary tumors 2022. Available from www.fda.gov/drugs/resources-information-approved-drugs/fda-disco-burst-edition-fda-approval-adstiladrin-nadofaragene-firadenovec-vncg-patients-high-risk.

30. USFDA. FDA D.I.S.C.O. Burst Edition: FDA approval of CARVYKTI (ciltacabtagene autoleucel) for the treatment of adult patients with relapsed or refractory multiple myeloma after four or more prior lines of therapy, including a proteasome inhibitor, an immunomodulatory agent, and an anti-CD38 monoclonal antibody 2022. Available from www.fda.gov/drugs/resources-information-appro ved-drugs/fda-disco-burst-edition-fda-approval-carvykti-ciltacabtagene-autoleu cel-treatment-adult-patients.

31. Jannsen. European Commission Grants Conditional Approval of CARVYKTI® (Ciltacabtagene Autoleucel), Janssen's First Cell Therapy, for the Treatment of Patients with Relapsed and Refractory Multiple Myeloma 2022. Available from www.janssen.com/european-commission-grants-conditional-approval-carvykti-cil tacabtagene-autoleucel-janssens-first.

32. USFDA. FDA Approves First Gene Therapy to Treat Adults with Hemophilia B 2022. Available from www.fda.gov/news-events/press-announcements/fda-appro ves-first-gene-therapy-treat-adults-hemophilia-b.

33. EMA. Hemgenix: Authorisation details 2022. Available from www.ema.europa.eu/ en/medicines/human/EPAR/hemgenix#authorisation-details-section.

34. Technology P. FDA approves bluebird bio's Skysona to treat cerebral adrenoleukodystrophy 2022. Available from www.fda.gov/vaccines-blood-biolog ics/skysona.

35. Blubirdbio. bluebird bio Receives EC Approval for SKYSONA™ (elivaldogene autotemcel, Lenti-D™) Gene Therapy for Patients Less Than 18 Years of Age With Early Cerebral Adrenoleukodystrophy (CALD) Without Matched Sibling Donor 2021. Available from https://investor.bluebirdbio.com/news-releases/news-release-details/bluebird-bio-receives-ec-approval-skysonatm-elivaldogene.

36. USFDA. Stratagraft 2021. Available from www.fda.gov/vaccines-blood-biologics/ stratagraft.

37. USFDA. Rethymic 2021. Available from www.fda.gov/vaccines-blood-biologics/ rethymic.

38. EMA. Breyanzi: Authorization Details 2022. Available from www.ema.europa.eu/ en/medicines/human/EPAR/breyanzi#authorisation-details-section.

39. USFDA. FDA D.I.S.C.O. Burst Edition: FDA approval of Breyanzi (lisocabtagene maraleucel) for second-line treatment of large B-cell lymphoma 2022. Available from www.fda.gov/drugs/resources-information-approved-drugs/fda-disco-burst-edition-fda-approval-breyanzi-lisocabtagene-maraleucel-second-line-treatment-large-b.

40. USFDA. FDA Approves First Cell-Based Gene Therapy for Adult Patients with Multiple Myeloma 2021. Available from www.fda.gov/news-events/press-announcements/fda-approves-first-cell-based-gene-therapy-adult-patients-multiple-myeloma.

41. EMA. Abecma: Authorization Details 2021. Available from www.ema.europa.eu/en/medicines/human/EPAR/abecma#authorisation-details-section.

42. USFDA. TECARTUS (brexucabtagene autoleucel) 2021. Available from www.fda.gov/vaccines-blood-biologics/cellular-gene-therapy-products/tecartus-brexucabtagene-autoleucel.

43. EMA. Tecartus (Brexucabtagene autoleucel) 2020. Available from www.ema.europa.eu/en/medicines/human/EPAR/tecartus#authorisation-details-section.

44. USFDA. Zolgensma 2019. Available from www.fda.gov/vaccines-blood-biologics/zolgensma.

45. EMA. Zolgensma (onasemnogene abeparvovec): Authorization Details 2020 Available from www.ema.europa.eu/en/medicines/human/EPAR/zolgensma#authorisation-details-section.

46. USFDA. HPC Cord Blood 2018. Available from www.fda.gov/vaccines-blood-biologics/cellular-gene-therapy-products/hpc-cord-blood-md-anderson-cord-blood-bank.

47. FDA. YESCARTA (axicabtagene ciloleucel) 2017. Available from www.fda.gov/vaccines-blood-biologics/cellular-gene-therapy-products/yescarta-axicabtagene-ciloleucel.

48. EMA. Yescarta: Authorization Details 2017. Available from www.ema.europa.eu/en/medicines/human/EPAR/yescarta#authorisation-details-section.

49. USFDA. LUXTURNA 2017. Available from www.fda.gov/vaccines-blood-biologics/cellular-gene-therapy-products/luxturna.

50. EMA. Luxturna: Authorisation Details 2018. Available from www.ema.europa.eu/en/medicines/human/EPAR/luxturna#overview-section.

51. USFDA. Kymriah (tisagenlecleucel) 2017. Available from www.fda.gov/vaccines-blood-biologics/cellular-gene-therapy-products/kymriah-tisagenlecleucel.

52. EMA. Kymriah: Authorisation Details 2017. Available from www.ema.europa.eu/en/medicines/human/EPAR/kymriah#authorisation-details-section.

53. USFDA. CLEVECORD (HPC Cord Blood) 2016. Available from www.fda.gov/vaccines-blood-biologics/cellular-gene-therapy-products/clevecord-hpc-cord-blood.

54. USFDA. HPC, Cord Blood - LifeSouth 2015. Available from www.fda.gov/vaccines-blood-biologics/cellular-gene-therapy-products/hpc-cord-blood-lifesouth.

55. USFDA. HPC, Cord Blood - Bloodworks 2016. Available from www.fda.gov/vaccines-blood-biologics/cellular-gene-therapy-products/hpc-cord-blood-bloodworks.

56. USFDA. MACI (Autologous Cultured Chondrocytes on a Porcine Collagen Membrane) 2016. Available from www.fda.gov/vaccines-blood-biologics/cellular-gene-therapy-products/maci-autologous-cultured-chondrocytes-porcine-collagen-membrane.

57. USFDA. IMLYGIC 2015. Available from https://fda.gov/vaccines-blood-biologics/cellular-gene-therapy-products/imlygic.

58. USFDA. ALLOCORD (HPC Cord Blood) 2013. Available from www.fda.gov/vaccines-blood-biologics/cellular-gene-therapy-products/allocord-hpc-cord-blood.

59. USFDA. HPC, Cord Blood 2012. Available from www.fda.gov/vaccines-blood-biologics/cellular-gene-therapy-products/hpc-cord-blood.

60. USFDA. DUCORD (HPC Cord Blood) 2012. Available from www.fda.gov/vaccines-blood-biologics/cellular-gene-therapy-products/ducord-hpc-cord-blood.

61. USFDA. GINTUIT (Allogeneic Cultured Keratinocytes and Fibroblasts in Bovine Collagen) 2012. Available from www.fda.gov/vaccines-blood-biologics/cellular-gene-therapy-products/gintuit-allogeneic-cultured-keratinocytes-and-fibroblasts-bovine-collagen.

62. USFDA. HEMACORD (HPC, cord blood) 2011. Available from www.fda.gov/vaccines-blood-biologics/cellular-gene-therapy-products/hemacord-hpc-cord-blood.

63. USFDA. LAVIV 2011. Available from www.fda.gov/vaccines-blood-biologics/cellular-gene-therapy-products/laviv.

64. USFDA. Provenge 2010. Available from www.fda.gov/vaccines-blood-biologics/cellular-gene-therapy-products/provenge-sipuleucel-t.

65. Drago D, Foss-Campbell B, Wonnacott K, Barrett D, Ndu A. Global regulatory progress in delivering on the promise of gene therapies for unmet medical needs. Molecular Therapy - Methods & Clinical Development. 2021;21:524–9.

66. Alvaro D. Quality and Regulatory Challenges Surrounding New Cell and Gene Therapy Products: PHARMA'S ALMANAC. Available from www.pharmasalmanac.com/articles/quality-and-regulatory-challenges-surrounding-new-cell-and-gene-therapy-products.

67. Lanucara F. Addressing the unique regulatory challenges of gene therapies. Available from www.biopharma-excellence.com/articles/addressing-the-unique-regulatory-challenges-of-gene-therapies/.

68. ICH. Mission: Harmonisation for Better Health. Available from www.ich.org/page/mission.

69. Mullin T. International regulation of drugs and biological products. In: Gallin JI, Ognibene FP, Johnson LL, editors. Principles and Practice of Clinical Research. 2018. p. 87–98.

70. Fusaroli M, Isgrò V, Cutroneo P, Ferrajolo C, Cirillo V, Del BF, et al. Post-marketing surveillance of CAR-T-cell therapies: analysis of the FDA Adverse Event Reporting System (FAERS) Database. Drug Safety. 2022;45(8):891–908.

71. Enrico F, Magdi E, Michaela S, Spencer PH, Mohamed A-E-E. Post-marketing safety and efficacy surveillance of cell and gene therapies in the EU: a critical review. Cell & Gene Therapy Insights. 2019;5(11):1505–21.

Index

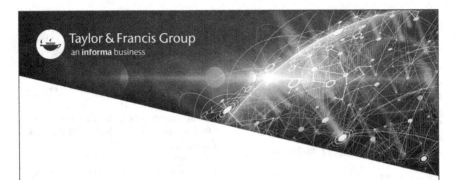

Printed in the United States
by Baker & Taylor Publisher Services

Printed in the United States
by Baker & Taylor Publisher Services